the g.i. diet CLINIC

RICK GALLOP

Also by Rick Gallop

The G.I. Diet
Living the G.I. Diet
The G.I. Diet Guide to Shopping and Eating Out
The Family G.I. Diet
The G.I. Diet Cookbook

the g.i. diet CLINIC

RICK GALLOP

RANDOM HOUSE CANADA

www.randomhouse.ca

Library and Archives Canada Cataloguing in Publication

Gallop, Rick
    The G.I. diet clinic : Rick Gallop's week-by-week guide to permanent weight loss / Rick Gallop.

Includes index.

ISBN 978-0-679-31439-4

    1. Reducing diets. 2. Glycemic index. I. Title.
RM222.2.G3423 2007   613.2'5   C2007-903426-8

Printed and bound in Canada

10 9 8 7 6 5 4 3 2 1

To the thirty-five e-Clinic members, whose commitment, enthusiasm and honesty over the course of the twelve-month program made this book possible.

Contents

Introduction

Ever since I wrote the original *G.I. Diet* back in 2002, my mission has been to help as many people as possible lose weight and keep it off. It all began during my own personal struggle to lose weight. Though I had been working to raise awareness of heart disease and stroke as president of the Heart and Stroke Foundation of Ontario, and was earnestly promoting healthy lifestyle choices among Canadians to reduce their risk for those diseases, the sad truth was that I was overweight myself. In an effort to lose the extra pounds, I tried deprivation diet after starvation diet, weighed everything I put into my mouth, and calculated calories, points and carbs. But nothing I tried worked; I could never manage to lose more than a few pounds. It was so frustrating and demoralizing that if I hadn't felt duty-bound to walk the talk as the chief representative of the Heart and Stroke Foundation of Ontario, I may well have given up. But I knew how dangerous my habits were to my health, and I doggedly persevered.

When eventually I found a diet based on the principles of the glycemic index, or G.I., which measures the speed at which your body breaks down carbohydrates and converts them to glucose, the vehicle your body uses for energy, I miraculously lost the extra weight that had been plaguing me for so long. I realized that, while I'd been blaming myself and my lack of willpower, the real reason I hadn't been able to slim down was that I didn't have the right information. I felt compelled to help other people who were trying to lose weight.

I persuaded my friends and associates to try the diet as well. But by the end of twelve months, 95 percent of them had dropped out. I was so disappointed; I wanted to know why the diet hadn't worked for them. They gave two reasons: (1) The diet was too complicated to follow, requiring them to count grams and calculate formulas and ratios; and (2) they were always hungry. I felt that if I could solve these two fundamental problems, I could help people lose weight and improve their health. The result was *The G.I. Diet,* a nutritionally ideal way to eat that emphasizes fruits and vegetables, whole grains, low-fat dairy products, lean protein and the "best" fats. As you can see, the G.I. Diet doesn't eliminate any food groups. Its easy-to-follow colour-coded system means you will never have to count calories or points, or weigh and measure food. It will keep you feeling satisfied and energetic as you slim down to your ideal weight.

Since publication of *The G.I. Diet,* I've received tens of thousands of letters from readers thrilled with their weight loss. The diet proved so successful that word quickly spread, and to date over two million copies have been sold in seventeen languages in twenty-two countries.

Desperation is a major theme in the letters I receive. Many of them sound something like this: "I have struggled with my weight all my life and I've tried everything—Weight Watchers, Jenny Craig, Atkins, etc.—and despite some short-term success, I'm always back where I started, or worse. Help!" Those who have an above-average amount of weight to lose find they have an even harder battle. Their problem is not only the amount of weight they want to lose, but also their fear of failure and their low self-esteem. Virtually all have struggled with being overweight or obese for most of their lives, frequently since childhood. For them, food is a fickle friend: it gives them a short-term feeling of well-being and comfort, but soon undermines their health, appearance and self-confidence.

Given the additional challenges facing people with an above-average amount of weight to lose, I decided to run a special program through my website. I asked those who had a body mass index (BMI) of 33 or over—in other words, the clinically obese—to participate in an "e-Clinic." For thirteen weeks, I would send them a weekly e-mail introducing them to the basics of the G.I. Diet, teaching them how to shop, cook and eat out, coaching them through the hurdles and helping them develop strategies for dealing with cravings and the emotional reasons we eat. In return, participants would send me their measurements and a diary each week. At the end of the thirteen weeks—enough time for people to get a good grasp of the diet and feel committed to the program—we would switch to a monthly e-mail and diary.

Though hundreds of people applied, I could choose only forty to participate in the clinic. Remarkably, over 80 percent of these "hard cases" stuck with it until the end, and those who dropped out had to, for the most part, because of unrelated health problems. By the end of the first thirteen weeks, the average weight loss was an incredible 25 pounds! And I had received a wealth of feedback that I know will be tremendously helpful to others trying to achieve their weight-loss goals.

It's all here in *The G.I. Diet Clinic*. Part I explains the principles behind the G.I. Diet and how it works. Part II is the thirteen-week guide that will get you started and coach you through all the challenges and pitfalls of following a new way of eating. Each week's guide includes a meal plan, grocery list and excerpts from e-Clinic participants' diaries. You will find these comments, stories, stumbling blocks and achievements relevant to your own experiences.

At the end of the thirteen weeks, you will be invited to sign on for a further nine monthly e-mail letters that will provide the latest news on green-light products as well as recipes and tips. You will also be invited to submit your own monthly diary and measurements. The e-mail letters will also provide valuable updates on the experiences and progress of other e-Clinic members.

So if you have tried diet after diet with no success, then this is the proven program for you. Whether you have 30 or 130 pounds (or more) to lose, *The G.I. Diet Clinic* will lead you every step of the way toward losing those extra pounds and inches, and, as importantly, keeping them off.

PART I

The G.I. Diet

The Truth about Carbs, Fats and Protein

It's just about impossible to live in this country and not know that we are in the midst of an "obesity epidemic." If you watch television, listen to the radio, read the newspaper or simply notice the magazine headlines at the supermarket checkout, you can't help but be aware that nearly 56 percent of Canadians are overweight and that our obesity rate has doubled over the past twenty years. Everyone seems to have an explanation for our collective weight crisis: Some hold the fast-food industry responsible; others blame our sedentary lifestyle. Some maintain we are eating too much fat; others say we are eating too many carbohydrates. So what's the truth?

Well, all of these reasons are part of the answer. But if you reduce the problem to its physiological cause, it's actually quite simple: we're consuming more calories than we're expending, and the resulting surplus is stored around our waists, hips and thighs as fat. There's no mystery here. But to understand why we are consuming more calories, we need to get back to basics and look at the three fundamental elements of our diet: carbohydrates, fats and protein. We need to understand the role these components play in the digestive system and how they work together—whether we're in the process of getting fat or thin.

We'll start with carbohydrates, since the popularity of low-carbohydrate diets like the Atkins program has made them a hot topic and given them a bad rap. Carbohydrates have been so much in the news over the past few years that a new word—"carbs"—has entered the language. Though they've been blamed for all our weight problems, their role in weight control has really been misunderstood.

Carbohydrates

Carbohydrates are a necessary part of a healthy diet. They are rich in fibre, vitamins and minerals, including antioxidants, which we now know play an important role in the prevention of heart disease and cancer. Carbohydrates are also the primary source of energy for our bodies. They are found in grains, vegetables, fruits, legumes (beans) and dairy products.

Here is how carbs work: when you eat an orange or a bagel, your body digests the carbohydrates in the food and turns them into glucose, which provides you with energy. The glucose dissolves in your bloodstream and then travels to the parts of your body that use energy, such as your muscles and brain. So carbs are critical to everyone's health. When managing weight, however, it is important to realize that not all carbs are created equal.

Some carbohydrates break down into glucose in the digestive system at a slow and steady rate, gradually releasing their nutrients and keeping us feeling full and satisfied. Others break down rapidly, spiking our glucose levels and then disappearing quickly, leaving us feeling hungry again. For example, cornflakes and old-fashioned, large-flake oatmeal are both carbohydrates, but we all know the difference between eating a bowl of oatmeal for breakfast and eating a bowl of cornflakes. The oatmeal stays with you—it "sticks to your ribs," as my mother used to say—whereas your stomach starts rumbling an hour after eating the cornflakes, pushing you toward your next snack or meal. Throughout the course of a day, if you are eating carbs that break down rapidly, like cornflakes, as opposed to those that break down slowly, you will be eating more and, as a result, will begin to put on weight. If, however, you start eating carbs that break down slowly, like old-fashioned oatmeal, you will eat less and begin to lose weight. Selecting the right type of carb is key to achieving your optimum energy and weight. But how do you know which carbohydrate is the right type and which isn't?

Well, the first clue is the amount of processing that the food has undergone. The more a food is processed beyond its natural, fibrous state, the less processing your body has to do to digest it. The quicker you digest the food, the sooner you feel hungry again. This helps explain why the number of Canadian adults who are overweight has surged over the last fifty years. A hundred years ago, most of the food people ate came straight from the farm to the dinner table. Lack of refrigeration and scant knowledge of food chemistry meant that most food remained in its original state. However, advances in science, along with the migration of many women out of the kitchen and into the workforce, led to a revolution in prepared foods geared to speed and simplicity of preparation. The giant food companies—Kraft, Kellogg's, Del Monte, Nestlé, etc.—were born. We happily began spending more money for the convenience of prepared, processed, packaged, canned, frozen and bottled food. The Kraft Dinner era had begun.

It was during this period that the miller's traditional wind and water mills were replaced with high-speed steel rolling mills, which stripped away most of the key nutrients, including the bran, fibre and wheat germ (which could spoil), to produce a talcum-like powder: today's white flour. This fine white flour is the basic ingredient for most of our breads and cereals, as well as for baked goods and snacks such as cookies, muffins, crackers and pretzels. Walk through any supermarket and you will be surrounded by towering stacks of these flour-based processed products. And we're eating more and more of these foods; over the past three decades, our consumption of grain has increased by 50 percent. Our bodies are paying the price for this radical change in eating habits.

The second clue in determining whether a carbohydrate is the right type is the amount of fibre it contains. Fibre, in simple terms, provides low-calorie filler. It does double duty, in fact: it literally fills up your stomach, so you feel satiated; and your body takes much longer to break it down, so it stays with you longer and slows the digestive process. There are two forms of fibre: soluble and insoluble. Soluble fibre is found in carbs such as oatmeal, beans, barley and citrus fruits, and has been shown to lower blood cholesterol levels. Insoluble fibre is important for normal bowel function and is typically found in whole wheat breads and cereals, and most vegetables.

There are two other important components that inhibit the rapid breakdown of food in our digestive system, and they are fats and protein. Let's look at fats first.

Fats

Fat, like fibre, acts as a brake in the digestive process. When combined with other foods, fat becomes a barrier to digestive juices. It also signals the brain that you are satisfied and do not require more food. Does this mean that we should eat all the fat we want? Definitely not!

Though fat is essential for a nutritious diet, containing various key elements that are crucial to the digestive process, cell development and overall health, it also contains twice the number of calories per gram as carbohydrates and protein. If you decide to "just add peanut butter" to your otherwise disciplined regime, it doesn't take much of it—two tablespoons—to spike your total calorie count. As well, once you eat fat, your body is a genius at hanging onto it and refusing to let it go. This is because fat is how the body stores reserve supplies of energy, usually around the waist, hips and thighs. Fat is money in the bank as far as the body is concerned—a rainy-day investment for when you have to call up extra energy. This clever system originally helped our ancestors survive during periods of famine. The problem today is that we don't live with cycles of feast and famine—it's more like feast, and then feast again! But the body's eagerness for fat continues, along with its reluctance to give it up.

This is why losing weight is so difficult: your body does everything it can to persuade you to eat more fat. How? Through fat's capacity to make things taste good. So it's not just you who thinks that juicy steaks, chocolate cake and rich ice cream taste better than a bean sprout. That's the fat content of cake and steak talking.

Sorry to say, there's no getting around it: if you want to lose weight, you have to watch your fat consumption. In addition, you need to be concerned about the type of fats you eat; many fats are harmful to your health. There are four types of fat: the best, the good, the bad and the really ugly. The "really ugly" fats are potentially the most dangerous, and they lurk in many of our most popular snack foods. They are vegetable oils that have been heat-treated to make them thicken—the trans fats you've been hearing so much about in the media lately. They raise the amount of LDL, or bad, cholesterol in our bodies while lowering the amount of HDL, or good, cholesterol, which protects us from heart disease. As a result they boost our cholesterol levels, which thickens our arteries and causes heart attack and stroke. So avoid using trans fats, such as vegetable short-ening and hard margarine, and avoid packaged snack foods, baked goods, crack-ers and cereals that contain them. (You can spot them by checking labels for "hydrogenated" or "partially hydrogenated" oils.)

The "bad" fats are called saturated fats and almost always come from animal sources. Butter, cheese and meat are all high in saturated fats. There are a couple of others you should be aware of too: coconut oil and palm oil are two vegetable oils that are saturated and, because they are cheap, they are used in many snack foods, especially cookies. Saturated fats, such as butter or cheese, are solid at room temperature. They elevate your risk of heart disease and Alzheimer's. The evidence is also growing that many cancers, including colon, prostate and breast cancer, are associated with diets high in saturated fats.

The "good" fats are the polyunsaturated ones, and they are cholesterol free. Most vegetable oils, such as corn and sunflower, fall into this category. What you really should be eating, however, are the "best" fats, the monounsaturated fats, which actually promote good health. These are the fats found in olives, almonds, and canola and olive oils. Monounsaturated fats have a beneficial effect on chol-esterol and are good for your heart. This is one reason the incidence of heart dis-ease is low in Mediterranean countries, where olive oil is a staple. Although fancy olive oil is expensive, you can enjoy the same health benefits from less costly supermarket brands.

Another highly beneficial oil that falls into the "best" category is omega-3, a fatty acid found in deep-sea fish, such as salmon, mackerel, albacore tuna and herring, as well as in lake trout, walnuts, and flaxseed and canola oils. Some brands of eggs and liquid eggs also contain omega-3, which can help lower cholesterol and protect cardiovascular health.

So the "best" and "good" fats are an important part of a healthy diet and also help slow digestion. Still, they're fat and they pack a lot of calories. We have to be careful, then, to limit our intake of polyunsaturated fats when trying to lose weight.

Since protein also acts as a brake in the digestive process, let's look at it in more detail.

Protein

Protein is an absolutely essential part of your diet. In fact, you are already half protein: 50 percent of your dry body weight is made up of muscles, organs, skin and hair, all forms of protein. We need this element to build and repair body tissues, and it figures in nearly all metabolic reactions. Protein is also a critical brain food, providing amino acids for the neurotransmitters that relay messages to the brain. This is why it's not a good idea to skip breakfast on the morning of a big meeting or exam. The "brain fog" people experience on some diets is likely the result of diminished protein. Protein is literally food for thought.

The main sources of dietary protein come from animals: meat, seafood, dairy and eggs. Vegetable sources include beans and soy-based products such as tofu. Unfortunately, protein sources such as red meat and full-fat dairy products are also high in "bad," or saturated, fats, which are harmful to your health. It is important that we get our protein from sources that are low in saturated fats, such as lean meats, skinless poultry, seafood, low-fat dairy products, cholesterol-reduced liquid eggs, and tofu and other soy products. One exceptional source of protein is the humble bean. Beans are a perfect food, really: they're high in protein and fibre, and low in saturated fat. No wonder so many of the world's cuisines have found myriad wonderful ways to cook beans. North Americans need to become more bean savvy. Nuts are another excellent source of protein and are relatively low in fat—as long as you don't eat a whole bowlful.

Protein is much more effective than carbohydrates or fat at satisfying hunger. It will make you feel fuller longer, which is why you should try to incorporate some protein into every meal and snack. This will help keep you on the ball and feeling satisfied.

Now that we know how carbohydrates, fats and protein work in the digestive system, let's use the science to discover how to take off the extra pounds.

TO SUM UP

- Eat carbohydrates that have not been highly processed and that do not contain highly processed ingredients.
- Eat less fat overall and look for low-fat alternatives to your current food choices.
- Eat only monounsaturated and polyunsaturated fats.
- Include some protein in all your meals and snacks.
- Eat only low-fat protein, preferably from both animal and vegetable sources.

The Secret to Easy, Permanent Weight Loss

The "G.I." in G.I. Diet stands for glycemic index, which is the basis of this diet—and the only scientific phrase you'll need to know. The glycemic index is the secret to reducing calories and losing weight without going hungry. It measures the speed at which carbohydrates break down in our digestive system and turn into glucose, the body's main source of energy or fuel.

The glycemic index was developed by Dr. David Jenkins, a professor of nutritional sciences at the University of Toronto, when he was researching the impact of different carbohydrates on the blood sugar, or glucose, level of diabetics. He found that certain carbohydrates broke down quickly and flooded the bloodstream with sugar, but others broke down more slowly, only marginally increasing blood sugar levels. The faster a food breaks down, the higher its rating on the glycemic index, which sets sugar at 100 and scores all other foods against that number. These findings were important to diabetics, who could then use the index to identify low-G.I., slow-release foods that would help control their blood sugar levels. At right are some examples of the G.I. ratings of a range of popular foods.

Examples of G.I. Ratings			
High G.I.		Low G.I.	
Baguette	95	Orange	44
Cornflakes	84	All-Bran	43
Rice cake	82	Oatmeal	42
Doughnut	76	Spaghetti	41
Bagel	72	Apple	38
Cereal bar	72	Beans	31
Biscuit	69	Plain yogurt	25

What do these G.I. ratings have to do with the numbers on your bathroom scale? Well, it turns out that low-G.I., slow-release foods have a significant impact on our ability to lose weight. As I have explained, when we eat the wrong type of carb, a high-G.I. food, the body quickly digests it and releases a flood of sugar (glucose) into the bloodstream. This gives us a short-term high, but the sugar is just as quickly absorbed by the body, leaving us with a post-sugar slump. We feel lethargic and start looking for our next sugar fix. A fast-food lunch of a double cheeseburger, fries and a Coke delivers a short-term burst of energy, but by mid-afternoon we start feeling tired, sluggish and hungry. That's when we reach for "just one" brownie or bag of potato chips. These high-G.I. foods deliver the rush we want and then let us down again. The roller-coaster ride is a hard cycle to break. But a high-G.I. diet will make you feel hungry more often, so you end up eating more and gaining more weight.

Let's look at the other end of the G.I. index. Low-G.I. foods, such as fruits, vegetables, whole grains, pasta, beans and low-fat dairy products, take longer to digest, deliver a steady supply of sugar to our bloodstream and leave us feeling fuller for a longer time. Consequently, we eat less. It also helps that these foods are lower in calories. As a result, we consume less food and fewer calories, without going hungry or feeling unsatisfied.

The key player in this process of energy storage and retrieval is insulin, a hormone secreted by the pancreas. Insulin does two things very well. First, it regulates the amount of sugar (glucose) in our bloodstream, removing the excess and storing it as glycogen for immediate use by our muscles, or putting it into storage as fat. Second, insulin acts as a security guard at the fat gates, reluctantly giving up its reserves. This evolutionary feature is a throwback to the days when our ancestors were hunter-gatherers, habitually experiencing times of feast or famine. When food was in abundance, the body stored its surplus as fat to tide it over the inevitable days of famine.

A few years ago, I was on vacation in a remote part of central Mexico, visiting the Copper Canyon, which, incredibly, is larger and deeper than the Grand Canyon in Arizona. A tribe of Tarahumara Indians still resides there. Until recently, these indigenous peoples typically put on 30 pounds during the summer and fall, when the crops, particularly corn, were plentiful. Then, over the course of the winter, when food became scarce, they lost these 30 pounds. Insulin was the champion in this process, both helping to accumulate fat and then guarding its depletion.

Of course, food is now readily available to us at the nearest twenty-four-hour supermarket. But our bodies still function very much as they did in the earliest days. When we eat a high-G.I. food, our pancreas releases insulin to reduce the glucose level in our blood, which, if left unchecked, would lead to hyperglycemia. If we aren't using all that energy at the moment, the glucose is stored as fat. Soon we become hungry again. Our body can either draw on our reserves of fat and laboriously convert them back to sugar, or it can look for more food. Since giving up extra fat is the body's last choice—who knows when that supply might come in handy!—our body would rather send us to the fridge than work to convert fat back to sugar. This helped our survival back in the old days, but it gets in the way of weight loss now.

So our goal is to limit the amount of insulin in our system by avoiding high-G.I. foods, which stimulate its production, and instead choosing low-G.I. foods, which keep the supply of sugar in our bloodstream consistent. Slow-release, low-G.I. carbohydrates help curb your appetite by leaving you feeling fuller for a longer period of time. When you combine them with lean protein and the best fats, which help slow the digestive process, you have the magic combination that will allow you to lose weight without going hungry.

Translated into real food, what does this mean? Well, for dinner you could have a grilled chicken breast, boiled new potatoes, a side salad of romaine lettuce and red pepper dressed with a bit of olive oil and lemon juice, and some asparagus if you feel like it. The trick is to stick with foods that have a low G.I., are low in fat and are low-ish in calories. This sounds—and is, in fact—quite complex. It might seem to you as though I'm breaking my promise of an easy weight-loss plan. But don't worry: I've done all the calculations, measurements and math for you, and sorted the foods you like to eat into one of three categories based on the colours of the traffic light. On pages 285–295, you will find the Complete G.I. Diet Food Guide, which has a list of foods in a red column, a list in a yellow column, and a list in a green column. Here's how the colour-coded categories work:

Red-Light Foods

The foods in the red column are to be avoided. They are high-G.I., higher-calorie foods that will make it impossible for you to lose weight.

Yellow-Light Foods

The foods in the yellow column are mid-range G.I. foods that should be treated with caution. They should be avoided when you are trying to lose weight, but once you've slimmed down to your ideal weight, you can begin to enjoy yellow-light foods from time to time.

Green-Light Foods

The green column lists foods that are low-G.I., low in fat and lower in calories. These are the foods that will allow you to lose weight. Don't expect them to be tasteless and boring! There are many delicious and satisfying choices that will make you feel as though you aren't even on a diet.

If you're a veteran of the low-carbohydrate craze, you'll be surprised to find potatoes and rice in the green-light column, but they are fine as long as they are the right type. Baked potatoes and french fries have a high G.I., while boiled new potatoes have a low G.I. The short-grain, glutinous rice served in Chinese and Thai restaurants is high-G.I., while long-grain, brown, basmati and wild rice are low. Pasta is also a green-light food—as long as it is cooked only until al dente (with some firmness to the bite). Any processing of food, including cooking, increases a food's G.I, since heat breaks down starch capsules and fibre, giving your digestive juices a head start. This is why you should never overcook vegetables; instead, steam them or boil them in a small amount of water just until they are tender. This way, they will retain their vitamins and other nutrients, and their G.I. rating will remain low.

While eating green-light foods is really the core of the G.I. Diet, there are a few more things you'll need to know to follow the program. Let's discuss these in the next chapter.

TO SUM UP
- Low-G.I. foods take longer to digest, so you feel satiated longer.
- The key to losing weight is to eat low-G.I., low-calorie foods—in other words, foods from the green-light column of the Complete G.I. Diet Food Guide.

The G.I. Diet Essentials

The G.I. Diet consists of two phases. For those with a more serious weight problem, an additional Preliminary Phase has been added. The Preliminary Phase and Phase I are the dramatic parts of the G.I. Diet—the period when those extra unwanted pounds come off! During these stages, you'll focus on eating foods that are low-G.I. and also low in fat and sugar—the foods in the green-light column of the Complete G.I. Diet Food Guide on pages 285–295. Yes, this means a farewell to bagels and a fond adieu to Häagen-Dazs. But it doesn't mean you won't have a multitude of delicious foods to choose from. Once you've slimmed down to your ideal weight, you enter Phase II, the maintenance phase of the program, which is the way you will eat for the rest of your life.

To decide whether you will be starting with the Preliminary Phase or Phase I, you will need to find out your body mass index (BMI), which is a measurement of how much body fat you are carrying relative to your height.

Your BMI

While the BMI gives a relatively accurate measure of body fat, it applies only to people who are twenty to sixty-five years of age. It isn't valid for children, pregnant or nursing women, the elderly or heavily muscled athletes. For the rest of us, however, it is the only accepted international standard for weight.

You can calculate your BMI from the table on pages 22–23 by running your finger down the left vertical column of the table until you reach your height. Then run your finger across that row until you find the number that is closest to your weight. The bold number at the top of that column is your BMI.

If your BMI falls between 19 and 24, your weight is within the acceptable norm and is considered healthy. Anything between 25 and 29 is considered overweight; if you're 30 or over, you are officially obese. **If your BMI is 32 or under**, I recommend you begin with Phase I of the program. If it's over 32, then start with the Preliminary Phase.

The Preliminary Phase and Phase I

Now that you know whether you'll be starting with the Preliminary Phase or Phase I, it's time to get into the details: what to eat, how much and how often.

What Do I Eat?

As you know, during the Preliminary Phase and Phase I, you will be sticking to the foods listed in the green-light column of the Complete G.I. Diet Food Guide on pages 285–295. To get a breakdown of your green-light choices for each meal, turn to pages 25–27, 30–32, 34–36 and 40.

How Much Do I Eat?

Remember, this is not a starvation diet—far from it. Going hungry is simply not necessary for weight loss; in fact, it's something to be resolutely avoided! Hunger is the absolute death knell for any weight-loss program. If you are hungry for a sustained period of time, your body will feel that it hasn't received enough fuel to meet its needs and will slow the rate at which it burns calories, making it even harder to lose those extra pounds. So never leave your digestive system with nothing to do. If your digestive system is busy processing food and steadily supplying energy to your brain, not only will your metabolism keep firing at a steady rate, but you won't be looking for high-calorie snacks. This is why you can, for the most part, eat as much green-light food as you want on the G.I. Diet.

In Phase I, you should be eating three meals and three snacks every day. And in the Preliminary Phase, you should be eating three meals and four snacks every day. The reason I recommend an extra snack in the Preliminary Phase is that someone with a larger body requires more calories just to keep functioning on a daily basis than someone who is lighter. This is also why I suggest larger serving sizes for some green-light foods in the Preliminary Phase than in Phase I. Although I generally do not restrict quantities of green-light foods—within reason (five heads of cabbage is a bit extreme)—there are a few exceptions, which I outline below. (Except where indicated, a serving size is per meal, not per day.)

Green-Light Servings

GREEN-LIGHT FOOD	PRELIMINARY PHASE (BMI OF 33 OR MORE)	PHASE I (BMI OF 32 OR LESS)
Crispbreads (with high fibre, e.g., Wasa Fibre)	3 crispbreads	2 crispbreads
Green-light breads (which have at least $2\frac{1}{2}$ to 3 grams of fibre per slice)	2 slices per day	1 slice per day
Green-light cereals	$\frac{2}{3}$ cup	$\frac{1}{2}$ cup
Green-light nuts	12 to 15	8 to 10
Margarine (non-hydrogenated, light)	3 teaspoons	2 teaspoons
Meat, fish, poultry	6 ounces	4 ounces (about the size of a pack of cards)
Olive/canola oil	$1\frac{1}{2}$ teaspoons	1 teaspoon
Olives	6 to 8	4 to 5
Pasta	1 cup cooked	$\frac{3}{4}$ cup cooked
Potatoes (new, boiled)	4 to 5	2 to 3
Rice (basmati, brown, long-grain)	$\frac{3}{4}$ cup cooked	$\frac{2}{3}$ cup cooked

BMI	19	20	21	22	23	24	25	26	27	28	29	30	31
	NORMAL						OVERWEIGHT					OBESE	
HEIGHT	WEIGHT (POUNDS)												
4'10"	91	96	100	105	110	115	119	124	129	134	138	143	148
4'11"	94	99	104	109	114	119	124	128	133	138	143	148	153
5'0"	97	102	107	112	118	123	128	133	138	143	148	153	158
5'1"	100	106	111	116	122	127	132	137	143	148	153	158	164
5'2"	104	109	115	120	126	131	136	142	147	153	158	164	169
5'3"	107	113	118	124	130	135	141	146	152	158	163	169	175
5'4"	110	116	122	128	134	140	145	151	157	163	169	174	180
5'5"	114	120	126	132	138	144	150	156	162	168	174	180	186
5'6"	118	124	130	136	142	148	155	161	167	173	179	186	192
5'7"	121	127	134	140	146	153	159	166	172	178	185	191	198
5'8"	125	131	138	144	151	158	164	171	177	184	190	197	203
5'9"	128	135	142	149	155	162	169	176	182	189	196	203	209
5'10"	132	139	146	153	160	167	174	181	188	195	202	209	216
5'11"	136	143	150	157	165	172	179	186	193	200	208	215	222
6'0"	140	147	154	162	169	177	184	191	199	206	213	221	228
6'1"	144	151	159	166	174	182	189	197	204	212	219	227	235
6'2"	148	155	163	171	179	186	194	202	210	218	225	233	241
6'3"	152	160	168	176	184	192	200	208	216	224	232	240	248
6'4"	156	164	172	180	189	197	205	213	221	230	238	246	254

BODY MASS

Source: U.S. National Heart, Lung and Blood Institute

INDEX (BMI)

		OBESE						EXTREMELY OBESE					
32	**33**	**34**	**35**	**36**	**37**	**38**	**39**	**40**	**41**	**42**	**43**	**44**	**45**
WEIGHT (POUNDS)													
153	158	162	167	172	177	181	186	191	196	201	205	210	215
158	163	168	173	178	183	188	193	198	203	208	212	217	222
163	168	174	179	184	189	194	199	204	209	215	220	225	230
169	174	180	185	190	195	201	206	211	217	222	227	232	238
175	180	186	191	196	202	207	213	218	224	229	235	240	246
180	186	191	197	203	208	214	220	225	231	237	242	248	254
186	192	197	204	209	215	221	227	232	238	244	250	256	262
192	198	204	210	216	222	228	234	240	246	252	258	264	270
198	204	210	216	223	229	235	241	247	253	260	266	272	278
204	211	217	223	230	236	242	249	255	261	268	274	280	287
210	216	223	230	236	243	249	256	262	269	276	282	289	295
216	223	230	236	243	250	257	263	270	277	284	291	297	304
222	229	236	243	250	257	264	271	278	285	292	299	306	313
229	236	243	250	257	265	272	279	286	293	301	308	315	322
235	242	250	258	265	272	279	287	294	302	309	316	324	331
242	250	257	265	272	280	288	295	302	310	318	325	333	340
249	256	264	272	280	287	295	303	311	319	326	334	342	350
256	264	272	279	287	295	303	311	319	327	335	343	351	359
263	271	279	287	295	304	312	320	328	336	344	353	361	369

Portions

Each meal and snack should contain, if possible, a combination of green-light protein, carbohydrates—especially vegetables and fruit—and fats. An easy way to visualize portion size is to divide your plate into three sections (see illustration below). Half the plate should be filled with vegetables; one-quarter should contain protein, such as lean meat, poultry, seafood, eggs, tofu or legumes; and the last quarter should contain a green-light serving of rice, pasta or potatoes.

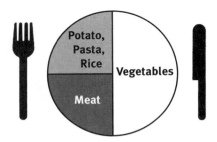

When Do I Eat?

Try to eat regularly throughout the day. If you skimp on breakfast and lunch, you will probably be starving by dinner and end up piling on the food. Have one snack mid-morning, another mid-afternoon and the last before bed. In the Preliminary Phase, the fourth snack can be eaten later in the afternoon if you usually have a late dinner, or during the evening if you generally have an early dinner. It's really up to you—have the extra snack at the time of day when you feel you most need it. The idea is to keep your digestive system happily busy so you won't start craving those red-light snacks.

Meal Basics

Because the green-light way of eating is most likely new to you, you're probably wondering what to eat instead of that bagel with cream cheese for breakfast, that hamburger for lunch, and those tortilla chips and salsa for a snack. On the following pages I'll go over your various green-light options for each of the main meals and snacks of your daily G.I. program. Let's start with breakfast.

Breakfast

I know you've been told that breakfast is the most important meal of the day, and it's actually true. It's the first thing you eat after your night-long "fast" of twelve hours or more, and it launches you into your workday. Eating a healthy breakfast will help you avoid the need to grab a coffee and Danish as soon as you hit the office, and will make you feel satisfied and energetic. Eating breakfast every day doesn't mean you have to set the alarm any earlier. If you have time to read the paper or feed the cat, you have time to prepare and eat a green-light breakfast.

The following chart lists typical breakfast foods in the colour-coded categories. To ensure you have a balanced breakfast, include some green-light carbohydrates, protein and fat. For a complete list of foods, see the Complete G.I. Diet Food Guide on pages 285–295.

Let's take a closer look at some of the usual breakfast choices.

PROTEIN			
Meat and Eggs	Regular bacon Sausages Whole regular eggs	Turkey bacon Whole omega-3 eggs	Back bacon Lean ham Liquid eggs/egg whites
Dairy	Cheese Cottage cheese (whole or 2%) Cream Milk (whole or 2%) Sour cream Yogurt (whole or 2%)	Cream cheese (light) Milk (1%) Sour cream (light) Yogurt (low-fat with sugar)	Buttermilk Cottage/cream cheese or sour cream (1% or fat-free) Extra low-fat cheese Fruit yogurt (non-fat with sugar substitute) Milk (skim) Soy milk (plain, low-fat)

CARBOHYDRATES

Cereals	All cold cereals except those listed as yellow- or green-light Granola Muesli (commercial)	Kashi Go Lean Crunch Kashi Good Friends Shredded Wheat Bran	All-Bran Bran Buds Fibre First Kashi Go Lean Oat Bran Porridge (old-fashioned rolled oats) Red River
Breads/Grains	Bagels Baguette Cookies Doughnuts Muffins Pancakes/Waffles White bread	Crispbreads (with fibre)* Whole-grain breads*	100% stone-ground whole wheat bread* Crispbreads (high fibre, e.g., Wasa Fibre)* Green-light muffins (see pp. 271–73) Whole-grain, high-fibre breads (2½–3 g fibre per slice)*
Fruits * Limit serving size (see page 21). ** For baking, it is OK to use a modest amount of dried apricots or cranberries.	Applesauce containing sugar Canned fruit in syrup Melons Most dried fruit	Apricots (fresh and dried)** Bananas Fruit cocktail in juice Kiwi Mango Papaya Pineapple	Apples Berries Cherries Grapefruit Grapes Oranges Peaches Plums

	Juices		
Juices	Fruit drinks Prune Sweetened juices Watermelon	Apple (unsweetened) Grapefruit (unsweetened) Orange (unsweetened) Pear (unsweetened)	Eat the fruit rather than drink its juice
Vegetables	French fries Hash browns		Most vegetables

FATS

	Butter	Most nuts	Almonds*
	Hard margarine	Natural nut butters	Canola oil*
	Peanut butter (regular and light)	Peanut butter (100% peanuts)	Hazelnuts*
	Tropical oils	Soft margarine (non-hydrogenated)	Olive oil*
	Vegetable shortening	Vegetable oils	Soft margarine (non-hydrogenated, light)*

* Limit serving size (see page 21).

Coffee and Tea

OK, this is the toughest one. The trouble with coffee is caffeine. It's not a health problem in itself, but it does stimulate the production of insulin. That's part of the "buzz" we get from coffee. But insulin reduces blood sugar levels, which then increases your appetite. Have you ever ordered a venti from Starbucks and then felt positively shaky an hour later? That's your blood sugar hitting bottom. You cure it by eating a bagel—which isn't helpful when you're trying to lose weight. So in Phase I, try to cut out caffeine altogether. As unpleasant as it may be, caffeine withdrawal will end in a day or two. Cut down gradually: go from a medium coffee to a small; then try a half-caffeinated, half-decaf blend. Then limit yourself to decaffeinated coffee—some brands taste as good as the real thing.

Even better, switch to tea. It has only about one-third of the caffeine that coffee has, and black tea and green tea have health benefits as well: they're rich in antioxidants, and beneficial for heart health and reducing the risk of dementia. Green tea is also considered an anti-carcinogen. (My ninety-seven-year-old mother and her tea-drinking cronies are living proof!) Herbal teas, such as peppermint, chamomile and other blends, are fine too, as long as they contain no caffeine.

If no coffee is going to be a deal breaker, then go ahead, have one cup a day—but not a double espresso. If you take milk and sugar, make it skim milk and a sweetener such as Splenda.

Cereals

Another toughie. Most cold cereals contain hidden or not-so-hidden sugars, and are therefore red-light. Green-light cereals are high in fibre; they have at least 10 grams per serving. All right, they're not a lot of fun by themselves, but you can liven them up with fresh, canned or frozen fruits, a few nuts and some fruit yogurt (fat-free, with sugar substitute).

My personal favourite cereal is good old-fashioned oatmeal—not the instant type that comes in packets but the large-flake, slow-cooking kind. (They're starting to serve it in the smartest hotels now.) Large-flake oatmeal is not only low-G.I., but also low calorie and has been shown to lower cholesterol. Yes, you have to cook it, but it takes only about three minutes or so in the microwave, and not much longer for one portion on the stovetop. Dress it up with yogurt, sliced almonds, berries or unsweetened applesauce. It's also just fine with nothing but milk on it.

I probably receive more e-mails about people's delight at rediscovering oatmeal than about any other food or meal. Give it a try.

Toast

Go ahead, but have no more than one slice per meal. Make sure your bread has at least 2½ to 3 grams of fibre per slice. (Note: Some bread labels quote a two-slice serving, which should equal 5 to 6 grams per serving.) The best choice is 100% stone-ground whole wheat bread, which has a coarser grind and therefore a lower G.I. White bread, cracked wheat or anything else made with white flour is red-light.

Butter and Jams

Butter is out. It's very high in saturated fat, and despite the protestations of the dairy industry, it's not good for your health or waistline. Yes, it does make things taste good—that's what fat does best. But you can still enjoy any one of a variety of light non-hydrogenated soft margarines, if you use only a teaspoon or so.

When buying fruit spreads, look for the "extra fruit/no sugar added" varieties. Fruit, not sugar, should be the first ingredient listed. These varieties taste great and don't have the calories of the usual commercial jams. Although I rarely plug brands, the President's Choice Blue Menu jams are a good buy.

Dairy

Low-fat dairy products are an ideal green-light choice and an excellent source of protein. I have a glass of skim milk every morning. I admit that skim didn't taste great at first, but I weaned myself off 2% by switching to 1% before moving on to skim. Now 2% tastes like cream!

Fat-free yogurt with sugar substitute instead of sugar is ideal for breakfast, dessert or a snack, either by itself or added to fruits or cereals. Low-fat cottage cheese is also a top-rated green-light source of protein. Or you can make a low-fat soft cheese spread by letting yogurt drain in cheesecloth overnight in the refrigerator.

Regular full-fat dairy products, including whole milk and cream, cheese and butter, are loaded with saturated fat and should be avoided completely.

Eggs

Use liquid eggs, such as Naturegg Break Free or Omega Pro. They are lower in saturated fat and cholesterol than regular eggs, and they make wonderful omelettes. Otherwise, use egg whites. If you're eating a hotel breakfast, in most cases the kitchen is happy to make omelettes with egg whites only.

Bacon

Bacon is red-light because of its high saturated-fat content. However, there are tasty green-light alternatives—such as Canadian back bacon, and lean ham— that make great BLTs.

Lunch

Lunch is usually the most problematic meal for my readers because they tend to eat it outside the home and in a hurry. Bringing your lunch to work is the easiest way to ensure you eat green-light. And there are other advantages to brown-bagging it, besides avoiding the temptation of a red-light lunch: it's cheaper, and it gives you downtime at your desk to read or catch up on paperwork. Here are the ground rules for making that brown bag a green-light bag. For a complete list of foods, see the Complete G.I. Diet Food Guide on pages 285-295.

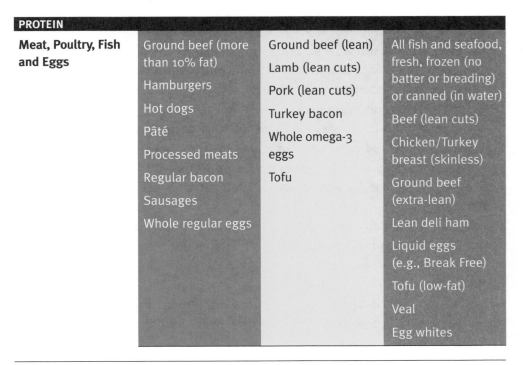

PROTEIN			
Meat, Poultry, Fish and Eggs	Ground beef (more than 10% fat)	Ground beef (lean)	All fish and seafood, fresh, frozen (no batter or breading) or canned (in water)
	Hamburgers	Lamb (lean cuts)	Beef (lean cuts)
	Hot dogs	Pork (lean cuts)	Chicken/Turkey breast (skinless)
	Pâté	Turkey bacon	Ground beef (extra-lean)
	Processed meats	Whole omega-3 eggs	Lean deli ham
	Regular bacon	Tofu	Liquid eggs (e.g., Break Free)
	Sausages		Tofu (low-fat)
	Whole regular eggs		Veal
			Egg whites

Breads/Grains			
Bagels	Crispbreads (with fibre, e.g., Ryvita High Fibre)	100% stone-ground whole wheat bread*	
Baguette/ Croissants	Pita (whole wheat)	Crispbreads (high fibre, e.g., Wasa Fibre)*	
Croutons	Tortillas (whole wheat)	Pasta (fettuccine, spaghetti, penne, vermicelli, linguine, macaroni)*	
Cake/Cookies	Whole-grain breads*	Quinoa	
Hamburger/ Hot dog buns		Rice (basmati, wild, brown, long-grain)*	
Macaroni and cheese		Whole-grain, high-fibre breads (2½– 3 g fibre per slice)*	
Muffins/Doughnuts			
Noodles (canned or instant)			
Pancakes/Waffles			
Pasta filled with cheese or meat			
Pizza			
Rice (short-grain, white, instant)			

Fruits/Vegetables			
Broad beans	Apricots	Apples	Carrots
French fries	Artichokes	Arugula	Cauliflower
Melons	Bananas	Asparagus	Celery
Most dried fruit	Beets	Avocado*	Cherries
Parsnips	Corn	Beans (green/wax)	Cucumbers
Potatoes (mashed or baked)	Kiwi	Bell peppers	Eggplant
Rutabaga	Mangoes	Blackberries	Grapefruit
	Papaya	Broccoli	Grapes
	Pineapple	Brussels sprouts	Leeks
	Potatoes (boiled)	Cabbage	Lemons
	Squash		Lettuce

* Limit serving size (see page 21).

	Red	Yellow	Green
Fruits/Vegetables		Sweet potatoes Yams	Mushrooms Olives* Onions Oranges (all varieties) Peaches Pears Peas Peppers (hot) Pickles Plums Potatoes (boiled new) Radishes Raspberries Snow peas Spinach Strawberries Tomatoes Zucchini

FATS

Red	Yellow	Green
Butter	Mayonnaise (light)	Almonds*
Hard margarine	Most nuts	Canola oil*
Mayonnaise	Peanut butter (100% peanuts)	Mayonnaise (fat-free)
Peanut butter (regular, light)	Salad dressings (light)	Olive oil*
Salad dressings (regular)	Soft margarine (non-hydrogenated)	Salad dressings (low-fat, low-sugar)
Tropical oils		Soft margarine (non-hydrogenated, light)*

SOUPS

Red	Yellow	Green
All cream-based soups	Canned chicken noodle	Chunky bean and vegetable soups (e.g., Campbell's Healthy Request, Healthy Choice)
Canned black bean	Canned lentil	
Canned green pea	Canned tomato	
Canned puréed vegetable		
Canned split pea		

* Limit serving size (see page 21).

Sandwiches

Sandwiches are a lunchtime staple, and it's no wonder: they're portable and easy to make, and they offer endless variety. They can also be a dietary disaster, but if you follow the suggestions below, you can keep your sandwiches green-light.

- Always use 100% stone-ground whole wheat or high-fibre whole-grain bread (2½ to 3 grams of fibre per slice).
- Sandwiches should be served open-faced. Either pack components separately and assemble just before eating or make your sandwich with a "lettuce lining" that helps keep the bread from getting soggy.
- Include at least three vegetables, such as lettuce, tomato, red or green bell pepper, cucumber, sprouts or onion.
- Instead of spreading the bread with butter or margarine, use mustard or hummus.
- Add up to 4 ounces of cooked lean meat or fish: roast beef, turkey, shrimp or salmon.
- If you make tuna or chicken salad, use low-fat mayonnaise or low-fat salad dressing and celery.
- Mix canned salmon with malt vinegar or fresh lemon.

Salads

Preparing salads may seem more labour intensive than making sandwiches, but it doesn't have to be. Invest in a variety of reusable plastic containers so you can bring individual-sized salads to work. Keep a supply of green-light vinaigrette on hand, and wash greens ahead of time and store in paper towels in plastic bags. You'll find that salads are a creative way to use up leftovers with a minimum of fuss.

Dinner

Dinner is traditionally is main meal of the day, and the one where we may have a tendency to overeat. We usually have more time for eating at the end of the day, and we generally feel fatigued as well, which encourages us to consume more. But since we will probably be spending the evening relaxing before going to bed, rather than being active, it is important that we don't overdo it. For a complete list of foods, see the Complete G.I. Diet Food Guide on pages 285–295.

The Protein

No dinner is complete without protein. Whether it is in the form of meat, poultry, seafood, beans or tofu, it should cover no more than one-quarter of your plate. A serving size should be 4 ounces,* which is roughly the size of the palm of your hand.

PROTEIN			
Meat, Poultry, Fish and Eggs	Breaded fish and seafood	Ground beef (lean)	All fish and seafood (not breaded or canned in oil)
	Fish canned in oil	Lamb (lean cuts)	
	Ground beef (more than 10% fat)	Pork (lean cuts)	Beef (lean cuts)
		Whole omega-3 eggs	Chicken breast (skinless)
	Hamburgers		
	Hot dogs		Ground beef (extra lean)
	Processed meats		Lean deli ham
	Sausages		Liquid eggs
	Sushi		Egg whites
	Whole regular eggs		Turkey breast (skinless)
			Veal
Dairy	Cheese	Cheese (light)	Cheese (fat-free)
	Cottage cheese (whole or 2%)	Milk (1%)	Cottage cheese/ sour cream (1% or fat-free)
	Milk (whole or 2%)	Sour cream (light)	
		Yogurt (low-fat)	
	Sour cream		Fruit yogurt (non-fat with sugar substitute)
	Yogurt (whole or 2%)		Milk (skim)
			Soy milk (low-fat)

* For Preliminary Phase servings see page 21.

Breads/Grains	Bagels	Pita (whole wheat)	100% stone-ground whole wheat bread*
	Baguette/Croissants	Whole-grain breads*	
	Cake/Cookies		Pasta (fettuccine, spaghetti, penne, vermicelli, linguine, macaroni)*
	Macaroni & cheese		
	Muffins/Doughnuts		
	Noodles (canned or instant)		Quinoa
	Pasta filled with cheese or meat		Rice (basmati, wild, brown, long-grain)*
	Pizza		Whole-grain, high-fibre breads (2 ½–3 g fibre per slice)*
	Rice (short-grain, white, instant)		
	Tortillas		
Fruits/ Vegetables	Broad beans	Apricots	Apples	Cherries
	French fries	Bananas	Arugula	Cucumbers
	Melons	Beets	Asparagus	Eggplant
	Most dried fruit	Corn	Avocado*	Grapefruit
		Kiwi	Beans (green/wax)	Grapes
	Parsnips	Mangoes		Leeks
	Potatoes (mashed or baked)	Papaya	Bell peppers	Lemons
		Pineapple	Blackberries	Lettuce
		Pomegranates	Broccoli	Mushrooms
		Potatoes (boiled)	Brussels sprouts	Olives*
		Squash		Onions
		Sweet potatoes	Cabbage	Oranges (all varieties)
			Carrots	
			Cauliflower	Peaches
		Yams	Celery	

* Limit serving size (see page 21).

Fruits/ Vegetables

		Pears
		Peas
		Peppers (hot)
		Pickles
		Plums
		Potatoes (boiled new)

		Radishes
		Raspberries
		Snow peas
		Spinach
		Strawberries
		Tomatoes
		Zucchini

FATS

Butter	Corn oil	Almonds*
Hard margarine	Mayonnaise (light)	Canola oil*
Mayonnaise	Most nuts	Hazelnuts
Peanut butter (regular, light)	Salad dressings (light)	Mayonnaise (fat-free)
Salad dressings (regular)	Soft margarine (non-hydrogenated)	Olive oil*
Tropical oils	Vegetable oils	Pistachios*
Vegetable shortening	Walnuts	Salad dressings (low-fat, low sugar)
		Soft margarine (non-hydrogenated, light)

SOUPS

All cream-based soups	Canned chicken noodle	Chunky bean and vegetable soups (e.g., Campbell's Healthy Request, Healthy Choice)
Canned black bean	Canned lentil	
Canned green pea	Canned tomato	
Canned puréed vegetable		Homemade soups with green-light ingredients
Canned split pea		

* Limit serving size (see page 27).

Red Meat

Though most red meat does contain saturated fat, there are ways to minimize it:

- Buy only low-fat meats such as top round beef. For hamburgers or spaghetti sauces, buy extra-lean ground beef. Veal and pork tenderloin are low in fat, too. As for juicy steaks, well, they are juicy because of the fat in them, so they're not a good choice.
- Trim any visible fat from the meat. Even a quarter inch of fat can double the total amount of fat in the meat.
- Broiling or grilling allows the excess fat from the meat to drain off. (Try one of those George Foreman–style fat-draining electric grills.)
- For stovetop cooking, use a non-stick pan with a little vegetable oil spray rather than oil. The spray goes further.

Poultry

Skinless chicken and turkey breast are excellent green-light choices. In the yellow-light category are skinless thighs, wings and legs, which are higher in fat.

Seafood

This is always a good green-light choice. Although certain cold-water fish, such as salmon and cod, have a relatively high oil content, this oil is omega-3 and is beneficial to your heart health. Shrimp and squid are fine, too, as long as they aren't breaded or battered. Fish and chips, alas, is out.

Beans (Legumes)

If you don't think you're into beans, it's time to re-evaluate! Beans are such an excellent source of so many good things: fibre, low-fat protein and "good" carbs that deliver nutrients while taking their time going through the digestive system. And they are a snap to incorporate into salads and soups to up the protein quotient. Chickpeas, lentils, navy beans, black beans, kidney beans—there's a bean for every day of the week. But watch out for canned pork and beans, which is high in sugar and fat, and avoid canned bean soups, which are processed to the point where their overall G.I. rating is too high. Homemade bean soups, however, are an excellent choice.

You will find several delicious recipes using beans in the recipes section of this book.

Tofu

You don't have to be a vegetarian to enjoy tofu, which is low in saturated fat and an excellent source of protein. While tofu is not necessarily a thriller on its own, it takes on the flavours of whatever seasonings and sauces it is cooked with. Seasoned tofu scrambles, for instance, are a good substitute for scrambled eggs. Choose soft tofu, which has up to one-third less fat than the firm variety.

Textured Vegetable Protein (TVP)

This is not a new device for pre-recording TV shows! TVP is a soy alternative to meat that looks a lot like ground beef, and can be used in the same ways—in lasagna, chili, stir-fries and spaghetti sauce. It's quite tasty and delivers the texture of meat. Our middle son, a vegetarian who has since left the nest, put us on to this adaptable product.

Potatoes, Pasta, Rice

These carbohydrates should cover only one-quarter of the plate. Remember, with potatoes your first choice is boiled small new potatoes. Most other choices, especially baked potatoes or french fries, are red-light. Sweet potatoes are a good lower-G.I. food, but since they tend to come in larger sizes, I suggest you save them for Phase II.

Your serving of pasta should be no more than 3/4 cup cooked*—just until al dente. If you have rice, make it 2/3 cup cooked basmati, wild, brown or long-grain rice.

* For Preliminary Phase servings see p.21.

Vegetables

Here you can put the measuring cup away. Eat as many vegetables and as much salad as you like; they should be the backbone of your meal. Always include at least two vegetables, and remember to cook them just until tender-crisp. Experiment with something you've never had before. Baby bok choy is delicious grilled, and rapini, a dark green vegetable that looks like broccoli with more leaves, is a nice change. The dark, curly green vegetables such as kale are full of good things, including folic acid.

Greens such as mesclun or baby spinach come conveniently pre-washed in bags. Frozen bags of mixed vegetables are also convenient and inexpensive; you can even toss the veggies into a saucepan, add tomato juice with a dollop of salsa and you have a quick vegetable soup.

Dessert

Yes, dessert is part of the G.I. Diet—at least, the kind that is green-light and good for you. This includes most fruits, and low-fat dairy products, such as yogurt and ice cream sweetened with sugar substitute rather than sugar. All my books have recipes for delicious green-light desserts.

Snacks

Keep your digestive system busy and your energy up with between-meal snacks—four a day during the Preliminary Phase and three a day during Phase I.

Try to eat balanced snacks that include a bit of protein and carbohydrates; for example, a piece of fruit with a few nuts, or cottage cheese with celery sticks.

A convenient snack for when you're on the go is half a nutrition bar. Be careful when choosing one: most are full of cereal and sugar. The ones to look for have 20 to 30 grams of carbohydrates, 12 to 15 grams of protein and 5 grams of fat. Balance and ZonePerfect bars are two examples.

Keep in mind that many snacks and desserts labelled "low-fat" or "sugar-free" aren't necessarily green-light. Sugar-free instant puddings and "low-fat" muffins are still high-G.I. because they contain highly processed grains.

SNACKS

Bagels	Bananas	Almonds**
Candy	Dark chocolate (70% cocoa)	Applesauce (unsweetened)
Cookies	Ice cream (low-fat)	Canned peaches/pears in juice or water
Crackers	Most nuts	
Doughnuts	Popcorn (air popped)	Cottage cheese (1% or fat-free)
Flavoured gelatin (all varieties)		Extra-low-fat cheese (e.g., Laughing Cow Light, Boursin Light)
French fries		
Ice cream		Fruit yogurt (non-fat with sugar substitute)
Muffins (commercial)		nutrition bars*
Popcorn (regular)		Hazelnuts**
Potato chips		Homemade green-light snacks (see pp. 270–75)
Pretzels		
Pudding		Ice cream (low-fat and no added sugar, e.g., Breyers Premium Fat-Free, Nestlé Legend)
Raisins		
Rice cakes		
Sorbet		
Tortilla chips		Most fresh fruit
Trail mix		Most fresh vegetables
White bread		Pickles
		Pumpkin seeds
		Sugar-free hard candies
		Sunflower seeds

* 180–225 calorie bars, e.g., ZonePerfect or Balance Bars; ¹/₂ bar per serving.

** Limit serving size (see page 21).

What Do I Drink?

Because liquids don't trip our satiety mechanisms, it's a waste to take in calories through them. Also, many beverages are high in calories. Juice, for example, is a processed product, and has a much higher G.I. than the fruit or vegetable it is made from. A glass of orange juice contains nearly two and a half times the calories of a fresh orange! So eat the fruit or vegetable rather than drink its juice. That way you'll get all the benefits of its nutrients and fibre while consuming fewer calories.

As well, stay away from any beverage that contains added sugar or caffeine. As I explained earlier, caffeine stimulates insulin, which leads to us feeling hungry. So no coffee or soft drinks containing caffeine in Phase I.

That said, fluids are an important part of any diet (I'm sure you're all familiar with the eight-glasses-a-day prescription). The following are your best green-light choices:

Water

The cheapest, easiest and best thing to drink is plain water. Seventy percent of our body consists of water, which is needed for digestion, circulation, regulation of body temperature, lubrication of joints and healthy skin. We can live for months without food, but we can survive only a few days without water.

Don't feel you have to drink eight glasses of water a day in addition to other beverages. Milk, tea and soft drinks all contribute to the eight-glasses-a-day recommendation. But do try to drink a glass of water before each meal—it will help you feel fuller so that you don't overeat.

Skim Milk

After a skeptical start, I've grown to really enjoy skim milk, and I like to drink it with breakfast and lunch, which tend to be a little short on protein. Skim milk is an ideal green-light food.

Soft Drinks

If you're used to drinking soft drinks, you can still enjoy the sugar- and caffeine-free diet ones. People often treat regular soft drinks and fruit juices as non-foods, but this is how extra calories slip by us.

Tea

Although black and green teas do contain caffeine, the amount is only about one-third of that of coffee. Tea has health benefits as well. Black and green teas contain antioxidant properties that help prevent heart disease and Alzheimer's. In fact, tea has more flavonoids (antioxidants) than any vegetable tested. Two cups of black or green tea have the same amount of antioxidants as 7 cups of orange juice or 28 cups of apple juice.

So tea in moderation is fine—minus the sugar and cream, of course. Try some new varieties: Darjeeling, Earl Grey, English Breakfast or spicy chai (with sugar substitute). Herbal teas, as long as they are caffeine-free, are also a green-light option, though they lack the flavonoids. Iced tea is acceptable if it's sugar-free.

Alcohol

Alcohol is generally a disaster for any weight-loss program. It puts your blood sugar on a roller coaster: you go up and feel great, then come down and feel like having another drink, or eating the whole bowl of peanuts. Alcohol also contains a lot of calories. So in Phase I, put away the corkscrew and the ice cube tray.

Now that you know how the G.I. Diet works, it's time to get ready to start. In the next chapter, I'll outline the steps for launching you into the program.

TO SUM UP
- In the Preliminary Phase and Phase I, eat only green-light foods.
- Eat three balanced meals plus four snacks a day in the Preliminary Phase and three balanced meals plus three snacks in Phase I.
- Pay attention to portion size: palm of your hand for protein, and a quarter plate for pasta, potatoes or rice. Use common sense and eat moderate amounts.
- Drink plenty of fluids, including an 8-ounce glass of water with meals and snacks (but no caffeine or alcohol).

Before You Start

The G.I. Diet it not so much a diet as a completely new and permanent way of eating. This is without question the most important message in this book. Unfortunately, most people view diets as a short-term change in eating habits that are ditched once weight loss targets have been achieved. They then revert to their old dietary habits and, not suprisingly, they are soon back at their original weight, or worse.

The G.I. Diet is the way you will eat for the rest of your life. The one constant refrain I received from the tens of thousands of successful readers is that this is a new way of eating that has become a permanent part of their lives.

Your motivation to lose weight is high, and with the G.I. Diet you now have the action plan that will help you make those unwanted pounds disappear. Still, to be successful you are going to have to make some significant changes in your life, and the better prepared you are, the better equipped you will be to handle any challenges that may arise. The following six steps will get you off to the best possible start.

1. Go see your doctor.

Before starting any major change in your eating patterns, check with your doctor to see if you have any health concerns that could affect your weight-loss plans. As you lose weight, your health will certainly improve, and it will be wonderfully motivating to learn that your blood glucose levels have improved or that your blood pressure has gone down. It may even be possible to change any medications you might be taking for weight-related conditions such as diabetes or high blood pressure.

2. Assess whether it's the right time to start.

Are you in the middle of a job change? A major house renovation or move? Is it the week before Christmas or before the cruise you've been planning for a year? Then it's probably not the best time to start a new way of eating. Some life events will make it harder—or even impossible—for you to give the program the attention it needs or to stick with it. Choose a period when your life is relatively stable and when you have time to learn new eating habits—not when your stress levels are even higher than usual. If your enthusiasm for a new slim you is high and the timing is right, then there's no better moment than the present!

3. Set your weight-loss target.

It's important to have a healthy, realistic weight-loss target in mind before starting the program. A good place to start is the BMI table on pages 22–23, not the glossy pages of a fashion or fitness magazine. Being too thin or too heavy is not good. Your health is at risk if your BMI is below 18.5 or above 25. As a woman, with a lower muscle mass and smaller frame than most men, you might want to target the lower end of the healthy range, say around 22, while men should generally target the higher end. Remember, the BMI tables are only a guide. Some of you, who have been carrying a significant amount of extra weight for a long time, will have developed a stronger skeletal frame and increased muscle mass to support this extra weight, and so a BMI in the low 20s would be unrealistic. If this is the case, you will want to target the higher end of the healthy range.

The other measurement you should concern yourself with is your waist measurement, which is an even better predictor of the state of your health than your weight. Abdominal fat is more than just a weight problem. Recent research has shown that abdominal fat acts almost like a separate organ in the body, except this "organ" is a destructive one that releases harmful proteins and free fatty acids, increasing your risk of life-threatening conditions, especially heart disease.

If you are female and have a waist measurement of 35 inches or more, or are male with a waist measurement of over 37 inches, you are at risk of endangering your health. Women with a measurement of 37 inches or more, and men with a measurement over 40 inches are at serious risk of heart disease, stroke, cancer and diabetes.

So I have your attention now! Make sure that you measure correctly: put a tape measure around your waist just above navel level till it fits snugly, without cutting into your flesh. Do not adopt the walking-down-the-beach-sucking-in-your-stomach stance. Just stand naturally. There's no point in trying to fudge the numbers, because the only person you're kidding is yourself.

Now that you know your BMI and waist measurement, you can set your weight-loss target and know roughly how long it will take you to reach that goal. When you lose weight in a healthy way, you can expect to lose about one pound per week. I say "about" because most people do not lose weight at a fixed and steady rate. The usual pattern is to lose more at the start of the diet, when you are losing mostly water weight, followed by a series of drops and plateaus. The closer you get to your target weight, the slower your weight loss will be. If you are planning to lose up to 20 percent of your body weight—for example, if you weigh 150 pounds and want to lose 30 pounds—assume this will take you thirty weeks, one pound per week. If you have more than 20 percent to shed, the good news is that you will lose at a faster rate. This is simply because your larger body weight requires more calories just to keep operating than someone who is lighter. Still, be prepared for measured results—it took you a while to put on those extra pounds and it will take some time to lose them. Be patient and know that once that weight is gone, it will be gone forever as you keep it off in Phase II of the program.

Although I recommend recording your progress, please don't get obsessed with numbers on the scale. Many people find themselves losing inches before they register any weight loss. Clothes start feeling a little looser, and before you know it you are down a dress size or getting into your old jeans. Soon you'll probably have to buy new clothes. My readers often tell me I should have warned them about the extra cost of refurbishing their closet!

4. Give your kitchen a green-light makeover.

Take a look in your fridge—what do you see? Two jars of mayonnaise, some left-over cheddar and a lot of sugar-laden condiments in jars? Now open the cupboards: what's the cookie and cracker situation? Now is the time to do an honest evaluation of what you tend to keep on hand. Consult the Complete G.I. Diet Food Guide (pages 205–295) and throw out anything that's in the red-light column. Be ruthless. If you always have chips on hand, you will eat them. If you keep Goldfish crackers around "for the kids," you can be sure that they won't be the only ones snacking on them. Give the unopened food items and cans to your skinny neighbours or local food bank.

5. Eat before you shop.

You know what happens when you drop by the supermarket on your way home from work, famished—before you know it you've bought the biggest tray of cannelloni ever made. The worst mistake you can make is to go shopping on an empty stomach. You'll only be tempted to fill your cart with high-G.I., sugar-rich foods.

6. Shop green-light.

For those of you who prefer a day-by-day guide to your planning, for each week of the G.I. Diet Clinic in Part II, I provide a complete meal and snack plan and a grocery list. If you'd rather not follow the plan, consult Chapter 3 to get some ideas of what you'd like to have for breakfast, lunch, dinner and snacks during your first week on the G.I. Diet; have a look at the Complete G.I. Diet Food Guide on pages 285–295; and peruse the recipe section of this book, *The G.I. Diet Cookbook,* or any of my other books. Write a shopping list and head out to the supermarket. Your first few green-light shopping trips will require a bit more time and attention than usual, as you familiarize yourself with green-light eating and meal planning. But don't worry: before long your new shopping and eating habits will become second nature.

Since it would be impossible to include every brand available in today's enormous supermarkets in the G.I. Diet Food Guide, I've listed categories of food rather than individual brands, except in cases where clarification is needed, or where there is an especially useful product available. This means that you will have to pay some attention to food labels when comparing brands.

When reading a food label, there are six factors to consider when making the best green-light choice:

Serving Size

Is the serving size realistic, or has the manufacturer lowered it to make the calories and fat levels look better than the competition's? When comparing brands, ensure that you are comparing the same serving size.

Calories

The product with the least amount of calories is obviously the best choice. Some products flagged as "low-fat" still have plenty of calories, so don't be fooled by the diet-friendly slogans. Calories are calories, whether they come from fat or sugar.

Fat

Look at the amount of fat, which is often expressed as a percentage, say 2 percent (good) or 20 percent (forget it). Then check to see what sort of fat it is. You want foods that are low-fat, with minimal or no saturated fats and trans fats. Remember that trans fats are often called "hydrogenated oils" or "partially hydrogenated oils."

Fibre

Foods with lots of fibre have a low G.I., so this is an important component. When comparing brands, choose the one with higher fibre.

Sugar

Choose products that are low in sugar. Again, watch for products advertised as "low-fat." Companies will sometimes quietly bump up the sugar content to make up for any perceived loss of taste. This often happens with yogurts and cereals.

Sugars are sometimes listed as dextrose, glucose, fructose or sucrose; regardless of the form, it's sugar.

Sodium

Sodium (salt) increases water retention, which doesn't help when you are trying to lose weight. It also contributes to premenstrual bloating in women and is a factor in hypertension (high blood pressure). Combine high blood pressure with excess weight and you move up to the front of the risk line for heart disease and stroke. Low-sodium products are therefore preferable.

The Recommended Dietary Allowance (RDA) for sodium is 2,500 mg, but this is generally regarded as too high. The U.S. National Academy of Science's new recommendation of 1,500 mg makes more sense. Since the average North American consumption of sodium per person per day is over 3,000 mg, it goes without saying that most of us could stand to cut back. However, if you have a BMI over 30 and have any blood pressure, circulation or heart problems, you need to be even more vigilant about seeking out low-sodium brands. Canned foods such as soups are often very high in sodium, as are many fast foods.

You've talked to your doctor, decided there's no better time than the present to lose weight and get healthy, set your weight-loss target, cleared your kitchen of fat-building foods, and restocked your pantry with delicious green-light choices. Now all you have to do is eat green-light meals and snacks each day and you're well on your way to your new trim self. In the next section, you'll find a week-by-week guide to all the challenges and issues that will come up as you follow the G.I. Diet for the first thirteen weeks. By the end of it you will know everything there is to know to achieve your weight-loss dreams, and you'll have lost a significant amount of weight along the way!

TO SUM UP

The six steps to get you launched into the G.I. Diet are:
1. Consult your doctor.
2. Assess whether it's the right time in your life to start.
3. Set your weight-loss target.
4. Give your kitchen a green-light makeover.
5. Eat before you shop.
6. Shop green-light.

PART II

The G.I. Diet Clinic

Week 1

Getting Started

Welcome to Week 1 of the G.I. Diet! You are starting on a journey, a new way of eating that will be the way you eat for the rest of your life. You will never have to go hungry or feel deprived. You won't have to count a calorie or a point. As long as you eat exclusively from the long list of green-light foods in the Complete G.I. Diet Food Guide, the extra weight will come off, and you will feel healthy and energetic eating the nutritious green-light way. No more yo-yo dieting! This is the way to lose weight permanently.

The first thing I would like you to do is fill in your current measurements below, as well as your target weight, so that you have a baseline with which to compare your progress and a place to remind yourself of your ultimate weight-loss goal. There is nothing more motivating than recording your success, so I will be asking you to write down your weight and waist and hip measurements at the end of each week. Be sure to weigh and measure yourself at the same time of day each week, since a meal or even a bowel movement can make a difference of a pound or two at a time when every pound counts! An ideal time is first thing in the morning, before breakfast.

Current Weight:_____

Current Waist:_____

Current Hips:_____

Target Weight:_____

Why Do You Want to Lose Weight?

Over the next thirteen weeks, I will be providing you with the knowledge, the tools and the counsel to help make this an easy and relatively painless transition to a new way of eating. But ultimately, for the program to work, you have to want to make it happen and you have to make the commitment to yourself. Whether you want to lose 10 pounds or 100, it's important to look at the reasons you want to lose weight. Your answer will have a lot to do with your motivation to start and, more important, stay the course with your new way of eating.

The following are some reasons e-Clinic participants gave for wanting to lose weight:

> "I am probably 100 pounds overweight, have high blood pressure, and am facing knee replacement surgery within the next two years. Time to get serious!" —Karen

> "I am a 49-year-old woman who is not aging well . . . I am always short of breath and my legs ache constantly. I was recently referred to a gastroenterologist because my blood work showed higher than normal liver enzyme counts. With a warning of the seriousness of a fatty liver, I left feeling so depressed . . . I am afraid now for my life." —Beverley

> "I have been heavy all my life . . . I remember the jokes and taunting, no proms, no dates . . . I am an emotional eater and food has always been my comfort in times of sorrow, distress or loneliness." —Kathy

> "I'm at a point in my life where I have to do something to reduce my weight and improve my health. Perimenopause is giving me some serious problems and I understand that extra weight changes hormone production (and many other things). I am quite certain that returning to an appropriate BMI would decrease the problems I'm having. It's affecting not only my life, but my children's lives, and I'm scared for their future. If our family lifestyle changes because I am changing mine, then so much the better. I want and need to do this." —Cecile

> "I am a nurse who should be looking healthy and promoting a healthy lifestyle. I know that the fat that is presently around my waist is not only unattractive but unhealthy. I know that my knees would appreciate me carrying less weight." —Marcia

"I am a blind person who has put on too much weight over the last few years. For many years I weighed 135 pounds. After the death of my parents, I found myself eating chocolate bars in the middle of the night after having numerous nightmares. The weight continued to increase and before I knew it, I am at the weight that I am now. My energy has declined and my old clothes don't fit right. I feel that just because one does not have any vision, that doesn't mean that one should look bad." —Name witheld

"I have always had a weight problem, though not to the extreme, but now as I am getting older I have noticed that my hips are sore and I don't have as much energy as I used to. Having four grandsons under five, I want to get myself in better shape to keep up with them." —Pam

"I know that you often read that one's appearance should not be the motivator, but it does help me to envision, this time next year, walking into a store and being able to buy a "regular-sized" dress for the holidays." —Bernadette

Actually, there is absolutely nothing wrong with appearance being a motivator to lose weight. In fact, it is one of the top reasons people want to slim down. Let's look at the three most common reasons people want to lose weight and see how they reflect your own.

1. I want to look better.

Judging from the correspondence I have received—20,000 e-mails and counting—the day when people discover that they have to dig out their "skinny" pants again is at least as rewarding as seeing the numbers fall on the scale. Most of us would rather shop for clothes that flatter and show off the body rather than resort to camouflage. It's a powerful motivator to walk into a room and hear a friend ask, "Have you lost weight? You look terrific." I've sold more books based on word of mouth—people asking G.I. Diet readers how they lost their weight— than through any other marketing strategy.

But losing weight is not just about trying to live up to unreachable, red-carpet standards of beauty or thinness; it's about feeling at ease in your body and liking what you see in the mirror. Weight loss boosts self-esteem and confidence, which in turn makes it easier to maintain new eating habits. It's amazing the difference the loss of just a few pounds can make, not only to how you look in your clothes but to how you feel about yourself.

2. I want to feel more energetic and less lethargic.

Perhaps what I hear about most frequently from readers, other than the thrill of losing pounds or going down a dress size, is the surge of energy that comes with a lighter, healthier body. Just the other day, I witnessed a dramatic demonstration of the kind of burden extra weight can be. My wife and I had just completed some house renovations to suit our empty-nest lifestyle, and as we were restoring some order, I asked Ruth to carry a couple of 20-pound dumbbells up a flight of stairs to my new workout room. She could get them only to the first-floor landing before she had to put them down again. "How do people who are 40 pounds overweight get around, let alone climb stairs?" she wondered. And 40 pounds of extra weight is not something you can just put down when you want to. Imagine the energy that goes into carrying those pounds! That's the energy that will be available to you again if you shed the excess weight.

Readers also tell me about the delight they experience when they find themselves able to exercise more and to enjoy activities they haven't participated in since their teens. If regaining your former energy and vitality is important to you, you'll receive constant motivation as your new, lighter body rejoices in its recently acquired freedom to run, swim, play squash, or engage in any activity you may have given up for "lack of energy."

3. I want to be healthier.

Although health may not be your primary reason for losing weight, it is ultimately the most important one. Excess weight and poor diet are by far the most critical factors in increasing your chances of developing major diseases that can either undermine your quality of life or drastically shorten it. These include heart disease, stroke, cancer, diabetes and Alzheimer's. Of course, genes play a role in your risk of these diseases too, but anyone who is overweight and undernourished is putting herself at increased risk for these conditions. The prospect of a long life, especially one free of pain, disability and disease, is a powerful motivator.

Below, I would like you to write down your own personal top three reasons for wanting to lose weight. Take a moment to be clear about your reasons, and be absolutely honest—this is for your eyes only. Later on, being able to come back to this page and read what you've written will go a long way toward keeping you motivated and helping you stick to your resolve.

My Top Three Reasons for Losing Weight

1. _____

2. _____

3. _____

Feeling a Little Nervous?

During the first week of the e-Clinic, everyone got off to an enthusiastic start. However, some participants felt a little trepidation:

"I am afraid and nervous because nothing has worked in the past and it all seems an impossibility now. However, I am committed and will take one day at a time." —Lynn

"I am anxious to start this new program. I look forward to the end result which is a slimmer me. I have attempted many other diets, but I have failed." —Pat

It's perfectly understandable if you're feeling anxious about whether you'll succeed on the G.I. Diet, particularly if you've tried and failed on diets before. But please, don't be nervous. I'd failed on many diets before slimming down with green-light foods, and I have a file of literally thousands of people who have had great success on the G.I. Diet because the program addresses the very reasons other diets fail. The fact is that most diets really don't work. Why? I'm sure the following explanations will be familiar to you.

Why Most Diets Don't Work

1. Most diets leave you feeling hungry, weak and deprived. You stagger through the day with a grumbling stomach, but sooner or later you cave and order a pizza with double cheese. Feeling perpetually hungry is the primary reason that people give up on a diet.

2. The diet is too complicated and time consuming to follow. You spend each day weighing and measuring food, calculating carbs or calories, and keeping food diaries. Perhaps this is fun initially, but then it all just becomes a burden. You're too busy to follow a diet that feels more like a math exam.

3. You feel bad. Many diets cut out essential nutrients, leaving you feeling lethargic and concerned about your health. Is it any wonder people give up?

Goals and Rewards

Feeling nervous about the challenges ahead could be related to the prospect of a long journey and a considerable amount of weight to lose. If so, set a series of mini-goals for yourself. Perhaps your first mini-goal could be to lose 20 pounds, or to break the 200-pound barrier, or even to eat perfectly green-light for an entire week.

Decide what your first mini-goal will be and what you will reward yourself with once you reach that goal: A pedicure or a massage? An evening out to a movie or that new book you've been wanting to read? Once you've reached that goal, give yourself a big pat on the back and the reward you promised yourself, and then set your next mini-goal. Setting smaller goals for yourself and reaching them will bolster your self-confidence and convince you of your ability to reach your target weight.

Suffering Withdrawal Symptoms?

During Week 1, a few participants reported feeling some unpleasant symptoms:

> "I am finding that I am having really bad headaches since I have stopped having coffee. Up until Saturday, I would have an extra-large coffee on the way to work. I was in horrible pain today." —Tammy

> "I find I am shaky and light-headed but I am not overly hungry. It is just an awful weak feeling. My hands actually shake and I feel sick. Could this be sugar withdrawal?" —Beverley

Any major change in eating patterns requires an adjustment period, particularly when those high-sugar, high-G.I. foods are suddenly dropped from the menu. The good news is that this period of adjustment will be short because the G.I. Diet is geared to stabilize blood sugar levels, preventing those sugar highs and lows that have been a principal contributor to your weight problems.

Getting through the first week will be the hardest part. Drinking just one cup of coffee a day can cause a dependence, as can caffeinated tea or soft drinks. When you suddenly put an end to your caffeine intake, you are likely to experience a headache, fatigue, a "blue" mood or irritability, and difficulty concentrating. While these symptoms will soon pass, you may want to gradually reduce your caffeine intake, replacing half your regular coffee with decaf, and then making the transition to decaf only. If you can't imagine life without your morning jolt of java, go ahead and have it, but make it just one cup a day, and use skim milk and sweetener rather than cream and sugar.

By the end of the first week you will begin to feel much better—even better than you did before you started the G.I. Diet, as Ross discovered: "I stopped drinking coffee and cut out all junk food and junk snacks. Once the withdrawal symptoms passed, I started to feel more energetic . . . I've lost 1 1/2 inches from my waist and butt, and 1 inch from my neck. A slightly different guy (second chin shrinking) looks back at me as I shave in front of the morning mirror . . . This program looks fantastic and realistic. For the first time ever, I feel I really can do this."

A week later, Beverley would write: "I feel much better than last week, when I wrote about the shakes and feeling weak. I actually wake up without a headache—something that has not happened in a long time."

Congratulate yourself for getting through the first week on the program, and record your measurements below. Also, take the time to write about your experiences and feelings this week. Diaries help reveal issues you might have to work on, ways of thinking that might be holding you back, and strategies that could work well for you.

Week 1 Weight: _____

Week 1 Waist: _____

Week 1 Hips:_____

Week 1 Diary

_____

_____

_____

_____

_____

_____

_____

_____

Week 1 Optional Meal Plan

Note: You are *not* required to use these weekly meal plans and shopping lists.
Feel free to pick and choose and make up your own green-light meals.

	BREAKFAST	SNACK	LUNCH	SNACK	DINNER	SNACK
MON	Homey Oatmeal (p. 204) with chopped apple	Cranberry Cinnamon Bran Muffin (p. 271)	Open face chicken sandwich with with lettuce, tomato and onion, and Basic G.I. Salad (p. 221)	Laughing Cow Light cheese with crispbread	Easy-Bake Lasagna (p. 237) and Caesar Salad (P. 222)	Mixed berries tossed in lime juice with sour cream
TUES	Mini Breakfast Puffs (p. 208)	Fruit yogurt	G.I. Pasta Salad (p. 225)	Hummus with carrot and celery sticks	G.I. Fish Fillet (p. 244), asparagus, carrots and new potatoes	Orange and almonds
WED	Homemade Muesli (p. 205) with skim milk and fruit yogurt	Cranberry Cinnamon Bran Muffin (p. 271)	1/2 whole wheat pita with canned light tuna, lettuce, tomato and cucumber, and Basic G.I. Salad (p. 221)	Babybel Gouda Lite cheese with crispbread	Chicken Curry (p. 252) and and Raita Salad (p. 219)	Apple Pie Cookie (p. 282), and glass of skim milk
THURS	Homey Oatmeal (p. 204) with blueberries	Small apple and glass of skim milk	Quick and Easy Chicken Noodle Soup (p. 216) and Basic G.I. Salad (p. 221)	Crunchy Chickpeas (p. 270)	Vegetable Crumble (p. 233), and Tabbouleh Salad (p. 226)	1/2 nutrition bar
FRI	All-Bran Buds with skim milk, peach slices and sliced almonds	Fruit yogurt	Mixed Bean Salad (p. 227)	Laughing Cow Light cheese with crispbread	Chicken Fried Rice (p. 251)	Mixed berries tossed in lime juice with sour cream
SAT	Western Omelette (p. 212)	1/2 nutrition bar	Greek Salad (p. 223)	Hummus with carrot and celery sticks	Beef and Eggplant Chili (p. 263) and Basic G.I. Salad (221)	Apple Pie Cookie (p. 282) and glass of skim milk
SUN	Oatmeal Buttermilk Pancakes with strawberries (p. 207)	Orange and almonds	Tuscan White Bean Soup (p. 215), and Basic G.I. Salad (p. 221)	Babybel Gouda Lite cheese with crispbread	Pork Medallions Dijon (p. 266), green beans, carrots and new potatoes	Piece of Plum Crumble (p. 278)

Week 1 Grocery List for Meal Plan

PRODUCE
Almonds (whole and sliced)
Apples
Asparagus
Baby spinach
Bean sprouts
Bell peppers (red and green)
Blueberries (fresh or frozen)
Broccoli
Carrots
Celery
Cranberries (dried)
Cucumbers (English and field)
Eggplant
Fresh herbs (chives, mint, flat-leaf parsley,
   sage, tarragon, thyme)
Garlic
Green beans
Green onions
Kale
Leeks
Lemons
Lettuce (iceberg, leaf and Romaine)
Mixed nuts
Mushrooms
Onions (yellow and red)
Oranges
Peaches (fresh or canned in juice or water)
Potatoes (new, small)
Prune plums (e.g., damson or Italian)
Raisins
Sesame seeds
Strawberries
Sunflower seeds, shelled and unsalted
Sweet potato
Tofu (firm)
Tomatoes (plum)
Zucchini

DELI
Feta cheese (light)
Hummus (light)
Kalamata olives
Parmesan cheese, grated

BAKERY
100% stone-ground whole wheat bread
Crispbread (e.g., Wasa Fibre)
Whole wheat pita bread

FISH COUNTER
Fish fillets (salmon or trout)

MEAT COUNTER
Back bacon
Chicken breasts (boneless, skinless)
Ground beef (extra-lean)
Pork tenderloins

**BEANS (LEGUMES) AND
CANNED VEGETABLES**
Chickpeas
Kidney beans (red and white)
Mixed beans
Diced tomatoes
Plum tomatoes
Tomato paste

PASTA AND SAUCES
Lasagna (whole wheat)
Rotini or penne (whole wheat)
Small pasta (e.g., ditali or tubetti)
Light tomato sauce (no added sugar)
Low-fat pasta sauce

SOUP AND CANNED SEAFOOD AND MEAT
Anchovy fillets
Chicken stock (low-fat, low-sodium)
Tuna (light, in water)
Vegetable stock (low-fat, low-sodium)

GRAINS AND SIDE DISHES
Basmati rice
Brown rice
Bulgur
Flaxseeds

INTERNATIONAL FOODS
Sesame oil
Soy sauce (low-sodium)
Tahini

COOKING OIL, VINEGAR, SALAD DRESSINGS AND PICKLES
Dijon mustard
Mayonnaise (fat-free)
Oil (canola and extra-virgin olive)
Red wine vinegar
Vegetable cooking oil spray (canola or olive oil)
Worcestershire sauce

SNACKS
Applesauce (unsweetened)
Nutrition bars (e.g., ZonePerfect, Balance Bar)

BAKING
Baking powder
Baking soda
Cornstarch
Oat bran
Spices (ground cardamom, cayenne pepper, chili powder, ground cinnamon, ground cumin, curry powder, ground ginger, ground nutmeg, dried oregano, black pepper, red pepper flakes, salt, dried thyme)

Splenda
Vanilla
Wheat bran
Wheat germ
Whole wheat flour

BREAKFAST FOODS
All-Bran Buds cereal
Oatmeal (large-flake oats)

BEVERAGES
White wine

DAIRY CASE
Babybel Gouda Lite cheese
Buttermilk
Cheddar cheese (low-fat)
Cottage cheese (1%)
Fruit yogurt (non-fat with sweetener)
Laughing Cow Light cheese (extra-low-fat)
Liquid eggs (e.g., Naturegg Break Free)
Milk (skim)
Mozzarella cheese (part-skim)
Plain yogurt (non-fat)
Soft margarine (non-hydrogenated, light)
Sour cream (low-fat)
Whole Omega-3 eggs

FROZEN FOODS
Mixed berries
Peas (or fresh)

Week 2

Meal Planning

This week I want to talk to you about meal planning and shopping. Setting some time aside each week to plan your meals and snacks for the seven days ahead is one of the most important things you can do to ensure that you eat well and stick to the program, as many of our e-Clinic participants discovered:

> "I've learned there is MUCH truth to the saying 'failing to plan is planning to fail.' In light of that, I prepared four selections from your cookbook last night to eat this week. Oh my goodness, the yogurt cheese with the sweetener and orange zest is fabulous! I made the almond-encrusted pears and put them (along with the yogurt cheese) on my oatmeal this morning . . . it was delicious. I also made the lentil and garbanzo bean salad, the chicken enchiladas, and the lentil and brown rice–stuffed peppers. So I'm going into the week prepared with some really yummy and healthy foods!" —Nancy

> "Well, I am embarrassed about what a bad week it has been. I was not prepared for many really busy days, and I have subsequently made poor choices daily. The whole week was just one problem perpetuating another. I have told you in the past that I do feel physically better when I make better food choices, but at a time when I needed as much energy as possible, I made the worst choices. So this week I am going to try a combination of better advance planning and writing down what I eat. I am trying not to feel too discouraged, as I really want to see success with this approach, but this week has shown me that determination alone is not sufficient if you don't make other changes also." —Bernadette

> "I had a much better week. Prior planning is the key so that snacks are ready and available. A shopping plan and list has solved this problem. Also brown-bagging it is so much easier. I bought an insulated nylon lunch bag with tons of room—works great." —Ross

> "I plan my meals in advance for a week, due to my long commute, and adjust as necessary." —Kathy

By and large, participants found that planning ahead was the key to their success on the program. If they neglected to do it, they tended to grab whatever happened to be easily available—and it usually wasn't green-light. Knowing what you are going to be eating each day and having all the ingredients at hand will not only ensure that you eat right, but also make your life simpler and put your mind at ease. This is why I have provided a green-light meal plan and shopping list for each week. I realize that some people enjoy cooking and trying new recipes, while others do not, and so these meal plans might not be practical for everyone. By the end of the thirteen weeks of the e-Clinic, Bernadette and Ross had found a meal-planning strategy that worked best for them:

> "For many weeks I struggled with the feeling that I had to start making full meals, and felt some (internal) pressure to start using recipes. But a simple approach to food preparation is working well for me and my family. The foods we are having may be somewhat plain by other people's standards, but so what? Fresh, homemade foods that are naturally tasty and colourful are working well for us. So we will stick to this for now." —Bernadette

> "I now work out a plan for a week or so, listing the days and the meals and a possible 'menu'—nothing fancy—for example, seven breakfasts, six lunches, and six dinners to cover before the next grocery trip. Then I calculate roughly what I will need for these meals by total breakfasts, lunches, dinners, snacks—not by specific days, that's far too anal for me. This takes only a few minutes to actually do the 'math' and write the list, plus, of course, I have to actually do the shopping. Say seven breakfasts equals oatmeal for five, high-fibre cereal for two, milk, sugar substitute, so many pieces of toast, jam, fruit, etc. I calculate what I want for this meal period and timeframe and buy what I need to bring the 'in home' stock up so I have no excuse to run out to Tim's because I need breakfast but don't have time to go shopping right now." —Ross

Decide what will work best for you in terms of meal planning and shopping, and then make your health a priority by following through.

Turning Your Standbys into Green-Light Recipes

You don't necessarily have to use all the recipes in this book; in fact, you can make many of your own standbys green-light by following the guidelines below.

Green-Light Ingredients

First, ensure that all the ingredients in the recipe are green-light. If there are any red- or yellow-light ingredients, either omit them or replace them with a green-light alternative. Some red- and yellow-light foods can be used in recipes if there is a very limited quantity, such as ½ cup of wine in a dish that will serve six people, or ¼ cup of raisins in a salad for four. Full-flavoured cheeses can also occasionally be used sparingly. For example, a tablespoon or two of grated Parmesan cheese sprinkled over a casserole will add flavour without too many calories. As long as the red- and yellow-light ingredients are used in limited quantities and not as a core ingredient, they will not have a significant impact on the overall G.I. or green-light rating of the recipe.

Fibre

The fibre content of the recipe is critical. Fibre, both soluble and insoluble, is key to the overall G.I. rating of a recipe. The more, the better. If your recipe is light on fibre, consider adding fibre boosters such as oats, bran, whole grains or beans.

Fat

The recipe should be low in fat with little to no saturated fat. If fat is called for, use vegetable oil. Canola and olive oil are your best choices, but use as little as possible, as all fats are calorie-dense.

Sugar

Never add sugar or sugar-based ingredients such as corn syrup or molasses. There are some excellent sugar substitutes on the market. My favorite is Splenda, or sucralose, which was developed from a sugar base but does not have as many calories. It works well in cooking and baking. Measure it by volume (not weight) to exactly replace sugar. For example, 1 tablespoon sugar = 1 tablespoon Splenda. Note that Brown Splenda is 50 percent sugar and is therefore not recommended.

Protein

Confirm that the recipe contains sufficient protein, or that you are serving it alongside some protein to round out the meal. Protein helps slow the digestive process, which effectively lowers the G.I. of a recipe. It is also the one component that is often overlooked, particularly in recipes for salads and snacks. Useful protein boosters are low-fat dairy products; lean meats, poultry and seafood; egg whites; beans; and soy-based foods, such as tofu and isolated soy or whey powders.

Maximizing the Time you Spend Cooking

If you don't always have time to cook, make big batches when you do have time, say on the weekends, and freeze green-light meals for busy nights. Having healthy meals in your freezer means you can always pull them out rather than grab a takeout menu. With a little preplanning, you won't have to rely on fast food to get you through your busy schedule! Organizing your pantry, fridge and freezer so that they keep you going when the going gets tough will ensure the weight-loss results you want, as Karen learned this week:

> "My weight is probably skewed because I have had bronchitis. Believe me, the combination of codeine, amoxicillin and cough drops is more effective than any diet I've ever been on! I am sure that once I get back to eating regularly my weight will go up, or at least I won't see any loss. Please remind me of this next week when I am discouraged. On the bright side, since I had already cleaned out my pantry and fridge, I didn't have my typical 'woe is me' feast of grilled cheese, tomato soup and chocolate ice cream/brownies." —Karen

Week 2 Weight: _____

Week 2 Waist: _____

Week 2 Hips: _____

Week 2 Diary

_____

_____

_____

_____

_____

_____

_____

_____

_____

_____

_____

_____

_____

Week 2 Optional Meal Plan

	BREAKFAST	SNACK	LUNCH	SNACK	DINNER	SNACK
MON	Homey Oatmeal (p. 204) with chopped apple	Carrot Muffin (p. 272)	Open-face lean deli ham sandwich with lettuce, tomato, red pepper and grainy mustard, and Basic G.I. Salad (p. 221)	Laughing Cow light cheese with crispbread	Fettuccine Primavera (p. 231), and Caesar Salad (p. 222)	Mixed berries tossed in lime juice with sour cream
TUES	Mini Breakfast Puffs (p. 208)	Fruit yogurt	Waldorf Chicken and Rice Salad	Hummus with carrot and celery	Ginger Wasabi Halibut (p. 246) Cold Noodle Salad with Cucumber and Sesame (p. 224), snow peas and carrots	Orange and almonds
WED	Homemade Muesli (p. 205) with skim milk and fruit yogurt	Carrot Muffin (p. 272)	Cottage cheese with apple and grapes, and Basic G.I. Salad (p. 221)	Babybel Gouda Lite cheese with crispbread	Chicken Tarragon with Mushrooms (p. 256), broccoli and basmati rice	Pecan Brownie (p. 294) and glass of skim milk
THURS	Homey Oatmeal (p. 204) with blueberries	Small apple and glass of skim milk	Minestrone Soup (p. 216) and Basic G.I. Salad (p. 221)	Crunchy Chickpeas (p. 270)	Meatloaf (p. 261), green beans, carrots and new potatoes	1/2 Nutrition bar
FRI	All-Bran Buds with skim milk, peach slices and sliced almonds	Fruit yogurt	1/2 whole wheat pita with deli turkey, lettuce, tomato and cucumber, and Basic G.I. Salad (p. 221)	Laughing Cow Light cheese with crispbread	Bean and Onion Pizza (p. 235)	Mixed berries tossed in lime juice with sour cream
SAT	Italian Omelette (p. 210)	1/2 nutrition bar	Crab Salad in Tomato Shells (p. 229)	Hummus with carrot and celery sticks	Grilled Tuna with Chimichurri Sauce (p. 247), asparagus and new potatoes	Pecan Brownie (p. 283) and glass of skim milk
SUN	Cinnamon French Toast (p. 206), with back bacon	Orange and almonds	Ham and Lentil Soup (p. 217), and Basic G.I. Salad (p. 229)	Babybel Gouda Lite cheese with crispbread	Orange Chicken with Almonds (p. 255), green beans and basmati rice	Slice of Apple Raspberry Coffee Cake (p. 279)

Week 2 Grocery List for Meal Plan

PRODUCE
Almonds (whole and sliced)
Apples
Asparagus
Baby spinach
Bell peppers (red and green)
Blueberries (fresh or frozen)
Broccoli
Carrots
Celery
Cucumbers (English and field)
Fresh herbs (basil, chives, cilantro, flat-leaf
    parsley)
Garlic
Ginger root
Grapes
Green beans
Green onions
Lemon
Lettuce (leaf and Romaine)
Limes
Mushrooms
Onions (yellow and red)
Oranges
Peaches (fresh or canned in juice or water)
Pecans
Potatoes (new, small)
Raisins
Raspberries
Sesame seeds
Snow peas
Strawberries
Sun-dried tomatoes
Sunflower seeds, shelled and unsalted
Tofu (firm)
Tomatoes (large beefsteak and plum)
Walnuts
Zucchini (yellow)

DELI
Feta cheese (light)
Hummus (light)
Lean deli ham
Lean deli turkey
Parmesan cheese, grated

BAKERY
100% stone-ground whole wheat bread
Crispbread (e.g., Wasa Fibre)
Whole wheat pita bread

FISH COUNTER
Frozen crab
Halibut fillets
Tuna steaks ($1/2$-inch thick)

MEAT COUNTER
Back bacon
Chicken breasts (boneless, skinless)
Ground beef (extra-lean)

BEANS (LEGUMES) AND CANNED VEGETABLES
Chickpeas
Kidney beans (red and white)
Lentils
Plum tomatoes
Tomato purée

PASTA AND SAUCES
Capellini or spaghettini (whole wheat)
Fettuccini or linguine (whole wheat)
Small pasta (e.g., ditali or tubetti)
Low-fat pasta sauce

SOUP AND CANNED SEAFOOD AND MEAT
Anchovy fillets
Chicken stock (low-fat, low-sodium)

Vegetable stock (low-fat, low-sodium)

GRAINS AND SIDE DISHES
Basmati rice
Flaxseeds

INTERNATIONAL FOODS
Mirin (or sweet sherry)
Rice vinegar
Soy sauce (low-sodium)
Sesame seeds (toasted)
Tahini
Wasabi powder

COOKING OIL, VINEGAR, SALAD DRESSINGS AND PICKLES
Buttermilk salad dressing (low-fat, low-sugar)
Dijon mustard
Grainy mustard
Oil (canola and extra-virgin olive)
Vegetable cooking oil spray (canola or olive oil)
Red wine vinegar
Worcestershire sauce

SNACKS
Nutrition bars (e.g., ZonePerfect, Balance Bar)

BAKING
Active dry yeast
Baking powder
Baking soda
Brown sugar substitute
Cornstarch
Oat bran
Spices (cayenne pepper, ground cinnamon, ground ginger, ground nutmeg, dried oregano, black pepper red pepper flakes, salt, dried tarragon, dried thyme)
Splenda
Unsweetened cocoa powder

Vanilla
Wheat bran
Wheat germ
Whole wheat flour

BREAKFAST FOODS
All-Bran Buds cereal
Oatmeal (large-flake oats)

BEVERAGES
Tomato juice
Vegetable cocktail juice
Vermouth or white wine

DAIRY CASE
Babybel Gouda Lite cheese
Buttermilk
Fruit yogurt (non-fat with sweetener)
Laughing Cow Light cheese (extra-low-fat)
Liquid eggs (e.g., Naturegg, Break Free)
Milk (skim)
Mozzarella cheese (part-skim)
Soft margarine (non-hydrogenated, light)
Sour cream (low-fat)
Whole omega-3 eggs

FROZEN FOODS
Peas (or fresh)
Mixed berries

Week 3

Behaviour Change

This week was clearly a period of adjustment as e-Clinic participants came to terms with the day-to-day realities of changing their eating habits:

> "Finishing things the kids have left on their plates has become such an established habit for me that there were times I was shocked to see myself on 'auto-pilot' just doing this, even when I wasn't hungry."
> —Bernadette

> "I had a good week but found that eating breakfast is the hardest thing for me to do. I am not really hungry, so I am choking down high-fibre cereal at my desk at seven in the morning. The weekend was better because I had time to make oatmeal, and you are right, it stays with you a lot longer than anything else." —Beverley

> "I found out that, for me, nuts can't be a snack. It is too easy to take a handful of cashews and almonds rather than the suggested amount, or to pop one or two extra as I count out the correct amount." —Kathy

> "I think where I went wrong this week was not eating enough small snacks. As a matter of fact, I often skipped the snacks, thinking that would help me in the long run . . . and more weight would be lost. Boy, I sure got fooled." —Pat

> "My problem is that I get really busy and forget to eat until I am starved and would eat any- and everything in my sight. I know this is not the way to be successful, but will work on eating and snacking at the right times." —Carol

> "Weekends are the hardest for me, as I don't have the structure of my workday with break time and lunch, so I may have to resort to a timer or alarm to remind me to eat. I usually end up not eating much at all throughout the day, then realizing I didn't eat very much and then having a slightly larger than normal dinner. I simply forget to

eat as I don't feel hungry—I get busy with doing things around the house or out and about and it doesn't occur to me to eat something." —Kimberley

Kimberley has an excellent idea there! If you are having trouble remembering to eat all your snacks and meals, why don't you buy a cheap watch with an alarm that you can set to remind yourself to eat. I have one myself for exactly that purpose, though of course it becomes unnecessary after a while when regular eating becomes second nature. Whatever you do, please don't forget to refuel! When you skip snacks or meals, you end up only eating more—not less—by day's end.

Breaking Bad Habits

Let's face it: change isn't always easy. Old habits can be hard to break. But to lose a significant amount of weight permanently, it is absolutely necessary to ditch old eating habits that led to the weight gain in the first place. Simply modifying your existing way of eating won't do it; you have to rethink your priorities and be willing to make fundamental changes in the way you approach food and eating. Making the commitment to commit is half the battle; making the necessary life changes is the rest. To ease the transition, bad habits will need to be replaced with good habits that you can easily handle. The following is a list of the top ten bad habits that prevent weight loss and what can be done to change them.

1. Skipping Breakfast

This is a very common bad habit: it is estimated that one-quarter of North Americans skip breakfast and the numbers are even worse for teenagers. A study of U.S. teens showed that only 32 percent were eating breakfast regularly!

Breakfast is the most important meal of the day. By the time people rise in the morning, most haven't eaten for ten to twelve hours, and their blood sugar levels are low. As a result, skipping breakfast will most certainly cause you to snack throughout the day in an effort to boost your blood sugar, or energy, level. And chances are good that you will reach for high-calorie, high-fat foods such as doughnuts, muffins or cookies to give you that quick sugar fix your body feels it needs. But as we are all well aware by now, the blood sugar high caused by these red-light foods will soon be followed by a sugar crash as your insulin kicks in, and you'll be looking for your next sugar fix.

It's tremendously important that you never skip breakfast. Research consistently shows that people who eat breakfast actually eat fewer calories per day and lose weight more successfully than those who do not. Always start your day with a substantial breakfast.

2. Not Taking Time to Eat Properly

Saying "I don't have time to eat properly" creates a spawning ground for bad habits. People who don't take the time to eat properly tend to grab a coffee and Danish on their way to work, eat a store-bought muffin mid-morning to boost flagging energy levels, have a slice or two of pizza with Coke for lunch, snack on chocolate and cookies in the afternoon to help keep their eyes open, pick up some high-fat takeout food on the way home for dinner, and finally collapse in front of the TV for the evening with beer and a bowl of pretzels.

It's easy to slip into this harmful cycle of fattening convenience foods and short-term energy fixes, but you'll pay for the convenience with a growing girth, flagging energy and poor health. And really, the amount of incremental time required to prepare your own healthy meals and snacks is quite modest. Fifteen minutes in the morning is all it takes to eat a healthy breakfast—often the length of time it takes to line up at Tim Hortons for a coffee. If you can't manage to wake up fifteen minutes earlier to squeeze in a nutritious breakfast before rushing off to work, then bring along a box of green-light cereal, a carton of skim milk and a piece of fruit. Another piece of fruit and a carton of skim milk takes no time to prepare and makes a filling, nutritious snack. And there are always places where you can get a green-light sandwich so you don't resort to pizza. Eating healthily throughout the day will ensure that you have the energy when you arrive home to prepare a quick green-light dinner in the time it would have taken to drive to the takeout place and wait for your order.

A little extra time and thought is all that's required to break out of the "I don't have time . . ." habits for good.

3. Grazing

The world's best grazers are teenagers. They simply cannot avoid opening the fridge every time they pass it. Their rapid growth and (hopefully) high activity levels require a constant high-calorie intake. Unfortunately, grazing is a habit that many people continue into their adult lives with disastrous results for their waistlines and health. A few nuts here, a couple of cookies there, a tablespoon or two of peanut butter, and a few glasses of juice all look pretty harmless in themselves, but taken together they can easily total several hundred extra calories a day! And those can add up to over twenty pounds of additional weight in a year.

On the G.I. Diet, you should be eating three meals plus three to four snacks a day, which means you are eating something approximately every two hours or so during your waking hours. This will reduce your temptation to graze. One reader wrote that she couldn't believe how she could be losing weight when she always seemed to be eating. She called it "green-light grazing"!

4. Unconscious Eating

How often have we all begun to nibble on a bowl of chips or nuts or a box of cookies while watching TV, reading a book or talking on the phone and then suddenly realized that we'd eaten the whole lot? Too often, I would guess.

Eating should never be the peripheral activity—it should always be the focus. Eat your meals at the table and set aside distractions such as the TV, computer, video game or telephone while you have your snacks. This will help you to always eat consciously and be aware of exactly how much you are eating.

5. Eating Too Quickly

The famous Dr. Johnson of the eighteenth century is said to have asserted that food should be always be chewed thirty-two times before swallowing. Though this seems rather excessive, there is an important truth here. Many of us tend to eat far too quickly. It takes twenty to thirty minutes for the stomach to let the brain know it is full. If you eat too quickly, you'll continue to eat past the point at which you've had enough. The solution, then, is to eat slowly to allow your brain to catch up with your stomach.

That's probably another reason Mediterranean countries have lower rates of obesity: they take far longer to eat their meals. There, mealtimes are for family and friends, and for enjoying the pleasure of food—not simply a means to tackle hunger. To ensure you are not eating more than your appetite requires, slow down and really enjoy what you are eating. Put your fork down between mouthfuls. Savour the flavours and textures.

6. Not Drinking Enough

Did you know that by the time you feel thirsty you are already dehydrated? Your body's need for water is second only to its need for oxygen. Up to 70 percent of the body is water, and we should be drinking about eight glasses a day to replenish our supply. Yet many of us don't take the time to drink enough, and we go through our days in a mild state of dehydration. Being dehydrated makes us feel tired and hungry, which makes us reach for food when really we should be reaching for a glass of water. Our body isn't hungry, it's thirsty. So always carry a water bottle with you and make sure you are drinking the recommended amount. Being properly hydrated will go a long way toward helping you control your appetite and lose weight.

7. Rewarding for Exercise

Another common habit is to reward yourself with food for doing some exercise. Rather than allowing the reward to lie in the exercise itself, many feel that the extra effort deserves some form of reward or treat, which more often than not takes the form of food or drink.

This raises a couple of issues. First, one of the great myths about weight loss is that it can be achieved through exercise. Though exercise is essential for long-term health and weight maintenance, it is actually a poor tool for losing weight. To give you an idea of how much exercise you would have to do to lose just one pound of fat, you would have to walk briskly for *forty-two* miles if you weighed 160 pounds or *fifty-three* miles if you weighed 130 pounds. That is a huge amount of effort and way beyond the capability or time availability of most people. Walking around the block or washing the car consumes only a handful of calories. So if you are using exercise as permission to cut a little slack in your diet, remember that that cookie reward will add more calories than you expended on your activity.

By all means exercise to improve your health, but don't think it will contribute a whole lot to your weight loss. I frequently tell people that losing weight is 90 percent diet and 10 percent exercise, particularly in the early stages.

8. Cleaning the Plate

Many of us were taught from the time we were small to finish what's on our plates before leaving the table. This becomes a deeply embedded habit that does not, unfortunately, help us in later life to lose or maintain weight. Not only do we finish our own, but we tend to also finish the leftovers on our children's plates or that last lonely slice in the pie dish after dinner. I confess that I do this. But this habit causes us to eat more than we need to satisfy our hunger and is therefore dreadful for weight control. Get into the habit of letting your stomach and brain decide when you are full, not the quantity of food on your plate. Leftovers can always be stored in the fridge, rather than around your waist and hips.

9. Shopping on an Empty Stomach

Human nature can often be perverse, encouraging us to do the right thing but at the wrong time. When you are full and satisfied, food shopping is rarely top of mind. But when you are hungry, grocery shopping suddenly seems like a very good idea indeed. Unfortunately, it just isn't: you'll end up with a shopping cart that has been filled primarily by your stomach rather than your head. Those red-light foods will seem far more tempting than usual, and you will probably make some poor choices as a result.

So always shop after a meal, or at least take a green-light snack, such as a portable muffin or nutrition bar, with you. You'll make far wiser choices this way.

10. Eating High-Sugar, High-Fat Treats

As we are all well aware, food is a big part of holidays and celebrations—just think of Thanksgiving, a wedding, a bar mitzvah or Christmas and you'll probably picture the special foods that go along with them. Where would the candy industry be without Valentine's Day, Halloween or Easter? Food is inexorably linked with positive experiences, and that is one reason we often think of certain foods as "treats." Whether it's Granny doling out candies to a child who has been good, or a neighbour presenting you with a freshly baked pie as reward for raking up her leaves, we are accustomed to using food treats to reward the people in our lives as well as ourselves. Unfortunately, these so-called treats tend to be high in calories, sugar and fat, and are certainly not your friends. They are a major contributor to the obesity crisis and to weight-related diseases such as diabetes and heart disease. We should really start to view these foods as penalties rather than rewards.

Instead choose treats that are lower in calories and fat. If candy is your thing, there is a plethora of low- and no-sugar brands available. Fresh fruit and low-fat, no-sugar-added yogurt and ice cream are even better treats. And there are many delicious green-light dessert and snack recipes in all my G.I. Diet books. Treats are a wonderful part of our lives—just make sure they are the right sort of treats.

Keep in mind that while it will take some effort and be challenging at times to change old bad habits, it's well worth your while to persevere with beneficial new behaviours. Before you know it, they'll be second nature, new habits as firmly entrenched as the old ones used to be. But these ones will help you slim down to a brand new you. To end this week on a positive note, here are some observations from e-Clinic participants as they completed week 3 of the program:

> "It's been a pretty good week . . . I've stayed totally on track with my eating, and feel SO much better physically (despite being sick) and have much more confidence in my ability to totally adapt to this lifestyle and get to my goal weight." —Nancy

"I feel more energetic for sure, and loose pants are still in fashion so I won't need new pants just yet." —Ross

"The weight is coming off so easily, I am really excited." —Tammy

Week 3 Weight: _____

Week 3 Waist: _____

Week 3 Hips: _____

Week 3 Diary

_____

_____

_____

_____

_____

_____

_____

_____

_____

_____

_____

Week 3 Optional Meal Plan

	BREAKFAST	SNACK	LUNCH	SNACK	DINNER	SNACK
MON	Homey Oatmeal (p. 204) with chopped apple	Apple Bran Muffin (p. 273)	Open-face chicken sandwich with lettuce, tomato and onion, and Basic G.I. Salad (p. 221)	Laughing Cow Light cheese with crispbread	Rigatoni with Mini Meatballs (p. 264) and Caesar Salad (p. 222)	Mixed berries tossed in lime juice with sour cream
TUES	Mini Breakfast Puffs (p. 208)	Fruit yogurt	G.I. Pasta Salad (p. 225)	Hummus with carrot and celery sticks	Citrus-Poached Haddock (p. 245), green beans and new potatoes	Orange and almonds
WED	Homemade Muesli (p. 205) with skim milk and fruit yogurt	Apple Bran Muffin (p. 273)	1/2 whole wheat pita with canned light tuna, lettuce, tomato and cucumber, and Basic G.I. Salad (p. 221)	Babybel Gouda Lite cheese with crispbread	Chicken Jambalaya (p. 254), and broccoli	Creamy Lemon Square (p. 284) and glass of skim milk
THURS	Homey Oatmeal (p. 204) with blueberries	Small apple and glass of skim milk	Quick and Easy Chicken Noodle Soup (p. 216) and Basic G.I. Salad (p. 221)	Crunchy Chickpeas (p. 270)	Barley Risotto with Leeks, Lemon and Peas (p. 232), and Tabbouleh Salad (p. 226)	1/2 Nutrition bar
FRI	All-Bran Buds with skim milk, peach slices and sliced almonds	Fruit yogurt	Mixed Bean Salad (p. 227)	Laughing Cow Light cheese with crispbread	Thai Red Curry Shrimp Pasta (p. 243)	Mixed berries tossed in lime juice with sour cream
SAT	Vegetarian Omelette (p. 211)	1/2 Nutrition bar	Greek Salad (p. 223)	Hummus with carrot and celery sticks	Zesty Barbecued Chicken (p. 258), Tangy Red and Green Coleslaw (p. 220), and new potatoes	Creamy Lemon Square (p. 284) and glass of skim milk
SUN	Oatmeal Buttermilk Pancakes (p. 207) with strawberries	Orange and almonds	Tuscan White Bean Soup (p. 215) and Basic G.I. Salad (p. 221)	Babybel Gouda Lite cheese with crispbread	Pork Tenderloin with Apple Compote (p. 268), Brussels sprouts, carrots and new potatoes	Piece of Berry Crumble (p. 277)

Week 3 Grocery List for Meal Plan

PRODUCE
Almonds (whole and sliced)
Apples
Bell peppers (red and green)
Blueberries (fresh or frozen)
Broccoli
Brussels sprouts
Cabbage (green and red)
Carrots
Celery
Cucumbers
Currants
Eggplant
Fresh herbs (chives, cilantro, flat-leaf parsley,
    mint, rosemary, sage and thyme)
Garlic
Green beans
Green onions
Kale
Leek
Lemons
Lettuce (leaf, iceberg and Romaine)
Limes
Mushrooms
Onions (yellow and red)
Oranges
Peaches (fresh or canned in juice or water)
Pecans
Potatoes (new, small)
Strawberries
Sunflower seeds, shelled and unsalted
Tomatoes (plum)
Zucchini

DELI
Feta cheese (light)
Hummus (light)

Kalamata olives
Parmesan cheese, grated

BAKERY
100% stone-ground whole wheat bread
Crispbread (e.g., Wasa Fibre)
Whole wheat pita bread

FISH COUNTER
Haddock fillets
Shrimp (large raw)

MEAT COUNTER
Chicken breasts (boneless, skinless)
Lean ground chicken or turkey
Pork tenderloin

BEANS (LEGUMES) AND CANNED VEGETABLES
Chickpeas
Kidney beans (red and white)
Mixed beans
Plum tomatoes
Stewed tomatoes
Tomato paste

PASTA AND SAUCES
Rotini or penne (whole wheat)
Marcaroni or small shells (whole wheat)
Rigatoni (whole wheat)
Spagettini or linguine (whole wheat)
Small pasta (e.g., ditali or tubetti)
Light tomato sauce

SOUP AND CANNED SEAFOOD AND MEAT
Anchovy fillets
Chicken stock (low-fat, low-sodium)
Tuna (light, in water)
Vegetable stock (low-fat, low-sodium)

GRAINS AND SIDE DISHES
Barley
Brown rice
Bulgur
Flaxseeds

INTERNATIONAL FOODS
Tahini
Thai red curry paste

COOKING OIL, VINEGAR, SALAD DRESSINGS AND PICKLES
Cider vinegar
Dijon mustard
Mayonnaise (fat-free)
Oil (canola and extra-virgin olive)
Red wine vinegar
Vegetable cooking oil spray (canola or olive oil)
Worcestershire sauce

SNACKS
Applesauce (unsweetened)
Nutrition bars (e.g., ZonePerfect, Balance Bar)

BAKING
Baking powder
Baking soda
Brown sugar substitute
Cornstarch
Ground almonds
Oat bran
Spices (ground allspice, bay leaves, cayenne pepper, celery seeds, chili powder, ground cinnamon, ground cloves, ground cumin, dried oregano, black pepper, dried sage, salt, dried thyme)
Splenda
Vanilla
Wheat bran

Wheat germ
Whole wheat flour

BREAKFAST FOODS
All-Bran Buds cereal
Oatmeal (large-flake oats)

BEVERAGES
Apple juice (unsweetened)
Dry white wine (or vermouth)

DAIRY CASE
Babybel Gouda Lite cheese
Buttermilk
Cheddar cheese (low-fat)
Fruit yogurt (non-fat with sweetener)
Laughing Cow Light cheese
Liquid eggs (e.g., Naturegg, Break Free)
Milk (skim)
Orange juice (unsweetened)
Soft margarine (non-hydrogenated, light)
Sour cream (low-fat)
Whole omega-3 eggs

FROZEN FOODS
Frozen apple juice concentrate
Mixed berries
Peas (or fresh)

Week 4

Falling off the Wagon

Falling off the wagon is bound to happen sooner or later. And while I don't encourage it, it's acceptable as long as it's the exception and not the rule. This diet isn't meant to be a straitjacket, after all. If you do your best to eat the green-light way 90 percent of the time, you'll still lose weight. The odd lapse, at worst, will delay you by a week or two from reaching your target weight. So don't be so hard on yourself; just get right back on the plan with the next meal. Some people make the mistake of feeling so bad about having a slip-up that they just give up. But you should anticipate that you will fall off the wagon from time to time. The best way to handle it is to learn why it happened and decide how you will handle the situation the next time. Rather than dwell on the negative, think about the positive, as Ross did: "There was a family dinner party with Chinese food where I strayed, but remarkably I only had one medium plate and not the usual two heaping plates of food I would have had in the past. Also, I felt no hunger pains when I didn't have the extra food this time—a definite change."

Here's how e-Clinic participants dealt with their occasional slip-ups:

> "Results, while unfortunate, were not unexpected. Two of the top three listed side effects of the prednisone I'm taking are increased appetite and weight gain. I've been eating a lot more. At home and the office, I've been limited to green-light foods, but the other day at a restaurant for lunch I found myself eating cornbread! I never eat cornbread. At least I didn't butter it. Two lessons from this week: (1) Keep green-light food handy and (2) the weight goes back on a whole lot easier than it comes off." —Karen

> "This past week has been really good, although I had a couple of functions where I couldn't follow the diet to the tee (I had a couple of alcoholic drinks and chicken strips with fries and ketchup). The next day, it was back to the diet. I felt extremely guilty, but my friends and family told me that it's okay to indulge once in a while, as long as I keep with my diet the rest of the time, which I do." —Tammy

"I had a little bump on Friday, when I went to a wedding that was a Henry VIII feast but still did way better than I would have had I not been thinking about what was going into my mouth."
—Beverley

"Last night I made a batch of cookies for a co-worker's birthday and was ridiculously hard on myself for eating ONE cookie. When I changed my perspective, however, I realized that just a few weeks ago I would've eaten about a dozen of those cookies and THEN beat myself up for having done so. Plus, eating that cookie made me think about trade-offs: would I rather eat the cookie or go off my plan in some other way, or would I prefer to use a bit of "wiggle room" to enjoy a glass of wine with dinner one night? There again, I can see that my perspective is changing, and that is of utmost importance for me to succeed, in my opinion." —Nancy

"The pull of a treat when life is stressful, or when you are on vacation or at a celebratory event can be so profound. I have come to learn over years of dieting, that if you slip up and make a bad choice, you need to get back on track ASAP, as one mistake can quietly transform into a week of mistakes. I think that process of reestablishing your focus must be critical in successful weight loss."
—Bernadette

Several participants said that the hardest part of the day was the evening, when they had the most difficulty steering clear of temptation. Some, like Ross, used green-light snacks to help them:

"I have my hardest time after work during prime snacking time, which was a major downfall period previously. I have put two of my snack times in here. I have managed to eat just green-light snacks, but some nights I still have cravings for the bad stuff. I feel like I imagine an alcoholic does on many nights."

Although most people find that their cravings do diminish after a few weeks on the G.I. Diet, because of the levelling effects that green-light eating has on one's blood sugar levels, there will be times when a craving will surface. Here's how to handle the situation:

1. Try to distract yourself with an activity. Call a friend, fold a basket of laundry, take out the garbage or just go for a walk. Sometimes a craving will pass.

2. If you're still having the craving, pinpoint the flavour you want and find a green-light food that has it. For example, if you want something sweet, have some strawberries or applesauce; if you want something sweet and creamy, try low-fat yogurt or ice cream with no added sugar; if you want something salty, have a couple of olives or a dill pickle, or some hummus with veggies; if it's chocolate you want, try half of a chocolate-flavoured nutrition bar or a mug of light instant chocolate. There are many green-light versions of the foods we normally reach for when a craving strikes.

3. Sometimes nothing but a piece of chocolate or a spoonful peanut butter will do. If this is the case, have a small portion and really enjoy it. Eat it *slowly* and savour the experience. Chalk it up to that 10 percent leeway you're allowed on the G.I. Diet. Just make sure you're staying green-light 90 percent of the time.

The good news is that as you continue with your green-light eating, you'll find yourself getting better and better at resisting those bad old foods. Have a look at what e-Clinic participants had to say:

"I'm finding the cravings diminishing since working on this diet, and driving by the fast-food places is less tempting as well. I'm encouraged that I can take more control over my eating, which is a relief to my wife!" —J

"Except for the one week I was away, plus the wedding, the weight is coming off. I keep expecting to get on the scale and see it's all a mistake. How is it possible to lose five pounds in one week? This has never happened in the past! Don't get me wrong, I'm pleased, but it seems like it's too good to be true." —Lynn

"It doesn't seem like I'm really on a diet (or doing a 'lifestyle change') in general. There are still the occasional times when I have a craving for a Hershey chocolate bar. During times like those, there is a yellow-light quick fix. That's when I'll take a small piece of my wife's organic 70 percent cocoa chocolate bar. It is just enough to take away the craving (the bitterness helps), and I stay on the green-light track the rest of the time." —J

Week 4 Weight: _____

Week 4 Waist: _____

Week 4 Hips: _____

Week 4 Diary

_____

_____

_____

_____

_____

_____

_____

Week 4 Optional Meal Plan

	BREAKFAST	SNACK	LUNCH	SNACK	DINNER	SNACK
MON	Homey Oatmeal (p. 204) with chopped apple	Whole Wheat Fruit Scone (p. 274)	Open-face lean deli ham sandwich with lettuce, tomato, red pepper and grainy mustard, and Basic G.I. Salad (p. 221)	Laughing Cow Light cheese with crispbread	Salmon Pasta (p. 242)	Mixed berries tossed in lime juice with sour cream
TUES	Mini Breakfast Puffs (p. 208)	Fruit yogurt	Waldorf Chicken and Rice Salad (p. 228)	Hummus with carrot and celery sticks	Pan-Seared White Fish with Mandarin Salsa (p. 248), broccoli, and basmati rice	Orange and almonds
WED	Homemade Muesli (p. 205) with skim milk and fruit yogurt	Whole Wheat Fruit Scone (p. 274)	Cottage cheese with apple and grapes, and Basic G.I. Salad (p. 221)	Babybel Gouda Lite cheese with crispbread	Chicken Schnitzel (p. 253), green beans, carrots and new potatoes	Slice of Strawberry Tea Bread (p. 275) and glass of skim milk
THURS	Homey Oatmeal (p. 204) with blueberries	Small apple and glass of skim milk	Minestrone Soup and Basic G.I. Salad (p. 221)	Crunchy Chickpeas (p. 270)	Mushroom and Gravy Pork Chops (p. 267), asparagus and basmati rice	1/2 nutrition bar
FRI	All-Bran Buds with skim milk, peach slices and sliced almonds	Fruit yogurt	1/2 whole wheat pita with deli turkey, lettuce, tomato and cucumber, and Basic G.I. Salad (p. 221)	Laughing Cow Light cheese with crispbread	Horseradish Burgers (p. 262) and Tabbouleh Salad (p. 226)	Mixed berries tossed in lime juice with sour cream
SAT	Back Bacon Omelette (p. 209)	1/2 nutrition bar	Crab Salad in Tomato Shells (p. 229)	Hummus with carrot and celery sticks	Vegetarian Moussaka (p. 239) and basmati rice	Slice of Strawberry Tea Bread (p. 275) and glass of skim milk
SUN	Cinnamon French Toast (p. 206) with back bacon	Orange and almonds	Ham and Lentil Soup (p. 217) and Basic G.I. Salad (p. 221)	Babybel Gouda Lite cheese with crispbread	Spicy Roasted Chicken with Tomatoes and Tarragon (p. 256), green beans and basmati rice	Slice of One-Bowl Chocolate Cake (p. 281) with berries

Week 4 Grocery List for Meal Plan

PRODUCE

Alfalfa sprouts (optional)
Almonds (whole and sliced)
Apples
Asparagus
Baby spinach
Bell peppers (red and green)
Blueberries (fresh or frozen)
Broccoli
Carrots
Celery
Cucumbers
Dried apricots
Eggplants
Fresh herbs (basil, chives, cilantro, flat-leaf
    parsley, mint, tarragon)
Garlic
Grapes
Green beans
Green onions
Lemons
Lettuce (leaf)
Limes
Mushrooms
Onions (yellow and red)
Oranges
Peaches (fresh or canned in juice or water)
Pecans
Potatoes (new, small)
Strawberries
Sun-dried tomatoes
Sunflower seeds, shelled and unsalted
Tomatoes (large beefsteak, plum, and cherry
    or grape)
Walnuts

DELI

Feta cheese (light)
Hummus (light)
Lean deli ham
Lean deli turkey
Light herb and garlic cream cheese
Parmesan cheese, grated

BAKERY

100% stone-ground whole wheat bread
Crispbread (e.g., Wasa Fibre)
Whole wheat breadcrumbs
Whole wheat hamburger buns
Whole wheat pita bread

FISH COUNTER

Frozen crab
Salmon fillet
White fish fillets

MEAT COUNTER

Back bacon
Boneless pork loin chops
Chicken breasts (boneless, skinless)
Ground beef (extra-lean)

BEANS (LEGUMES) AND CANNED VEGETABLES

Chickpeas
Kidney beans (red)
Lentils
Diced tomatoes
Plum tomatoes
Tomato paste

PASTA AND SAUCES

Macaroni (whole wheat)
Small pasta (e.g., ditali or tubetti)

SOUP AND CANNED SEAFOOD AND MEAT
Chicken stock (low-fat, low-sodium)

GRAINS AND SIDE DISHES
Basmati rice
Bulgur

INTERNATIONAL FOODS
Rice vinegar

**COOKING OIL, VINEGAR, SALAD
DRESSINGS AND PICKLES**
Buttermilk salad dressing (low-fat, low-sugar)
Dijon mustard
Grainy mustard
Horseradish
Mayonnaise (fat-free)
Oil (canola and extra-virgin olive)
Red wine vinegar
Steak sauce
Vegetable cooking oil spray (canola or olive
   oil)
Worcestershire sauce

SNACKS
Applesauce (unsweetened)
Nutrition bars (e.g., ZonePerfect, Balance Bar)
Canned mandarin oranges (no added sugar)

BAKING
Baking powder
Baking soda
Oat bran
Spices (ground allspice, dried basil, cayenne,
ground cinnamon, ground
   cumin, Italian herb seasoning, ground nut
   meg, dried oregano, black pepper, red pepper
   flakes, salt, dried thyme)
Splenda
Unsweetened cocoa powder

Vanilla
Wheat bran
Wheat germ
Whole wheat flour

BREAKFAST FOODS
All-Bran Buds cereal
Oatmeal (large-flake oats)

BEVERAGES
Apple juice (unsweetened)
Dry white wine (or vermouth)

DAIRY CASE
1% pressed cottage cheese
Babybel Gouda Lite cheese
Buttermilk
Fruit yogurt (non-fat with sweetener)
Laughing Cow Light cheese
Liquid eggs (e.g., Naturegg, Break Free)
Milk (skim)
Orange juice (unsweetened)
Soft margarine (non-hydrogenated, light)
Sour cream (low-fat)

FROZEN FOODS
Mixed berries
Peas (or fresh)

Week 5

Eating Out

It's high time we dealt with the tricky issue of eating out. I say tricky because, unlike when you eat at home, in restaurants you have little control over what goes into the meals and how they are prepared. Nevertheless, there are ways that you can minimize any potential damage, both in regular and in fast-food restaurants.

In restaurants, be especially aware of portion size. Over the past twenty years or so, there has been a dramatic increase in serving sizes—a phenomenon termed "portion distortion." Let me give you some examples from a list prepared by the U.S. National Heart, Lung and Blood Institute:

	TWENTY YEARS AGO		TODAY	
SNACKS				
	Size	**Calories**	**Size**	**Calories**
Bagel	3 inches	140	6 inches	350
French fries	2.4 ounces	210	7 ounces	610
Muffin	1.5 ounces	210	5 ounces	500
Cookie	1 1/2 inches	55	4 inches	275
MEALS	**Calories**			**Calories**
Spaghetti and meatballs	500			1025
Turkey sandwich	320			820
Chicken Caesar salad	390			700
Chicken stir-fry	435			865

As you can see, the size and corresponding calories of food have doubled or even tripled over a relatively short period. And we have come to accept these new supersized portions as standard. A study done with college students on their consumption of their favourite food, macaroni and cheese, shows that the more that was put in front of them, the more they ate. Yet they reported that they felt no fuller on the larger portions than on the smaller ones. Moral: if it's not on your plate, you won't miss it.

While these new supersizes may look like terrific value, just think what it has cost us in terms of extra pounds and poorer health. Difficult though it may be to refrain from eating everything that has been placed in front of you—I certainly suffer from this—moderation and common sense are your waistline's best friends. Don't feel guilty about leaving food on your plate! In addition to this fundamental recommendation, here are my top ten tips for dining out with family and friends the green-light way:

Top Ten Dining-Out Tips

1. Just before you go out, have a small bowl of high-fibre, green-light cold cereal (such as All-Bran) with skim milk and sweetener. I often add a couple of spoonfuls of no-fat/no-sugar fruit yogurt. This will take the edge off your appetite and get some fibre into your digestive system, which will help reduce the G.I. of your upcoming meal.

2. Once seated in the restaurant, drink a glass of water. It will help you feel fuller.

3. Remember to eat slowly to allow your brain the time it needs to realize you're full. Put your fork down between mouthfuls and savour your meal.

4. Once the basket of rolls or bread—which you will ignore—has been passed around the table, ask the server to remove it. The longer it sits there, the more tempted you will be to dig in.

5. Order a soup or salad first and tell the server you would like this as soon as possible. This will keep you from sitting there hungry while others are filling up on the bread. For soups, go for vegetable- or bean-based, the chunkier the better. Avoid any that are cream-based, such as vichyssoise. For salads, the golden rule is to keep the dressing on the side. Then you can use a fraction of what the restaurant would normally pour over the greens. Avoid Caesar salads, which come pre-dressed and often pack as many calories as a burger.

6. Since you probably won't get boiled new potatoes and can't be sure of what type of rice is being served, ask for double vegetables instead. I have yet to find a restaurant that won't oblige.

7. Stick with low-fat cuts of meat or poultry. If necessary, you can remove the skin. Duck is usually too high in fat. Fish and shellfish are excellent choices but shouldn't be breaded or battered. Tempura is more fat and flour than filling. Remember that servings tend to be generous in restaurants, so eat only 4 to 6 ounces (the size of a pack of cards) and leave the rest.

8. As with salads, ask for any sauces to be served on the side.

9. For dessert, fresh fruit and berries—without the ice cream—are your best choice. Most other desserts are a dietary disaster. My advice is to avoid dessert. If a birthday cake is being passed around, share your piece with someone. A couple of forkfuls or so along with your coffee should get you off the hook, with minimal dietary damage!

10. Order only decaffeinated coffee. Skim-milk decaf cappuccino is our family's favourite choice.

Fast Food

Not so long ago, the idea of getting a green-light lunch at a fast-food outlet was simply laughable. Now, however, partly due to the threat of legal action and a stagnant market share, the major fast-food chains are finally offering some healthy options. Subway has been pioneering the move toward healthy choices for some time, and its initiative has been reflected in its successful growth.

Although things are changing, fast food is still a minefield. Hamburgers are soaked in saturated fat, as are deep-fried chicken and fish. The trimmings—fries, ketchup, shakes and regular soft drinks—are loaded with fat and sugar.

While I normally recommend avoiding pizza restaurants like the plague, since pizza generally has high-G.I. crust and lots of saturated fat in the cheese toppings, Pizza Hut has made a real effort to improve its offerings. Your best bet there are the Thin 'N Crispy Pizzas and Fit 'N Delicious Pizzas, as well as garden salads and light dressings.

Below I've listed other good choices in fast food. An asterisk indicates items that are excessively high in sodium—the fast-food industry frequently boosts salt content when lowering fat to make up for any perceived loss of flavour—which can be hazardous to your health. Two asterisks indicate a stratospheric level of salt. (* = high salt content ** = extremely high salt content)

Ground Rules

1. Always eat burgers open-faced, throwing away the top half of the bun.
2. Always ask for low-fat dressings and use only half the sachet.

McDonald's

Salads
Chicken Oriental Salad

Dressings
Newman's Own Low Fat Balsamic Dressing*
Mild Chunky Salsa
Newman's Own Low Fat Sesame Thai Dressing*

Burgers and Sandwiches
Whole Wheat Chicken McGrill with BBQ Sauce*
Chicken Protein Platter*
McVeggie Burger*
Turkey BLT
Chicken Fajita (but only order one; two is over the line in fat and calories)

Snack
Fruit 'n Yogurt Parfait (hold the granola)

Wendy's

Salads
Mandarin Chicken Salad with Roasted Almonds
Spring Mix Salad with Honey Roasted Pecans

Dressings
Fat Free French Style
Reduced Fat Creamy Ranch
Low Fat Honey Mustard

Burgers and Sandwiches
Ultimate Chicken Grill Sandwich* plus side salad
Large Chili plus side salad

Snack
Junior Frosty (6-oz cup)

Burger King

Salads (hold the Garlic Parmesan Toast on all salads)
Fire-Grilled Chicken or Shrimp Caesar Salad
Fire-Grilled Chicken or Shrimp Garden Salad

Dressings
Ken's Honey Mustard Dressing
Ken's Border Ranch Salad Dressing

Burgers
BK Veggie Burger* plus side salad

Pizza Hut
See previous page

Harvey's

Salads
Entrée Grilled Chicken Caesar Salad
Entrée Grilled Chicken Garden Salad
Entrée Caesar Salad

Dressings
Light Caesar
Light Italian

Soups
Beef Barley*
Chicken Noodle*
Harvest Vegetable*

Burgers and Sandwiches
Grilled Chicken*
Veggieburger

Swiss Chalet

Meals (hold the flat bread)
Santa Fe Grilled Chicken Salad**
Vegetable Stir Fry on rice*
Chicken Stir Fry on rice**
Quarter Chicken Breast Dinner (skinless) with coleslaw, vegetables, or corn
Chicken on a Kaiser (white meat)

Dressings
Light Italian Dressing
No-Fat Raspberry Vinaigrette

Subway

Note: Best choice of roll is Italian or Wheat.

6-inch subs (with 6 grams of fat or less)

Roast Beef*
Oven Roasted Chicken
Turkey Breast*
Turkey Breast & Ham*
Veggie Delite
Sweet Onion Chicken Teriyaki*
Ham*

Deli-Style Sandwiches

Ham
Roast Beef
Turkey Breast

Salads

Veggie Delite (side salad)
Grilled Chicken & Baby Spinach

Dressings

Fat-Free Honey Mustard
Fat-Free Wine Vinaigrette
Fat-Free Sweet Onion

Tim Hortons

Note: Ask that your sandwich be made with a whole wheat bun.

Sandwiches

Garden Vegetable
Harvest Turkey Breast
Chicken and Roasted Red Pepper*

Soups

Tim's Own Chicken Noodle*
Vegetable Beef Barley*
Hearty Vegetable*
Turkey and Wild Rice*
Beef Noodle*
Chicken Gumbo*
Tomato Florentine*
Minestrone*

Note: This information was correct at time of publication. However, as this is a fast-changing marketplace, you may wish to check these restaurants' menus or websites from time to time to see if they have expanded their green-light offerings.

On the Road

Being away from home was a challenge for many in the e-Clinic. It is essential to plan ahead when travelling. When I am on the road during media tours, I frequently find myself in situations where there is no green-light food in sight. And these days on planes, there is often no food at all. I always carry emergency green-light reserves with me, such as nuts, nutrition bars (usually Balance Bars), homemade green-light muffins, and fruit.

Breakfast tends to be the biggest challenge of the day because I habitually eat breakfast where I'm staying, as most people do. (For lunch and dinner, there is usually a wider choice of venue and menu.) Fortunately, oatmeal appears to be increasingly available in hotels. Failing that, look for high-fibre cereals, yogurt and fruit. Skim milk is normally available on request. As a last resort, I always carry a couple of pouches of instant oatmeal with me, which requires only the addition of hot water. Though this option is not as good as large-flake oatmeal, it's certainly better than Sugar Pops!

If you can come to grips with snacks and breakfast, then staying green-light while travelling is definitely doable.

Here's how e-Clinic participants managed to stay in the green while eating out:

"I was away at a course on Thursday, Friday, Saturday and Sunday, and therefore making green-light choices was more difficult as I had no control of the food preparation! However, I am happy that all meals were served buffet-style, and therefore I was able to make the best of the situation by choosing vegetables and fruit, yogurt, some whole-grain bread, whatever protein wasn't covered by a sauce, etc., but this was tough at times as they had an amazing array of food at each break. (Do you know how many fruit trays are loaded with all the melons on the red-light list!) I did take a few things with me, like apples and almonds, so that if I needed a snack I had a decent choice on hand. I'm proud of myself that I was able to show restraint!" —Bernadette

"My toughest struggle this week was stadium food. I went to a soccer game. You really are at their mercy; they even check handbags on the way in (they say for security, but you aren't even allowed to bring in your own bottle of water). I had no problem skipping the beer, although usually over the course of the match I would have had two or three. The real problem was not so much craving bad food as the unavailability of anything the least bit healthy. I ended up getting a chicken burrito, begging a fork off another vendor, unwrapping the tortilla and eating the chicken, beans, tomatoes and some of the rice. You would think with all the media focus on obesity and healthy eating, someone would open up a salad bar or at least do grilled (as opposed to fried) chicken sandwiches. Maybe there's an opportunity for my second career." —Karen

"My experience eating regular food at the retreat was really good. I took small amounts of some of the food and left bread and desserts alone. I had cheese sticks, almonds and apples to eat in between meals, which kept me from being as hungry at mealtime. I allowed myself one treat: homemade cinnamon rolls. I was really surprised when I came home and had lost weight!" —Diane

"Eating out is still the biggest challenge. I went to a birthday party at East Side Mario's. It is almost impossible to find green-light food there, except for the salad, which I ate generously (dressing on the side and only a little used)." —Lynn

"I was in Toronto for four days last week for meetings and training. Because of time constraints, it was decided that we would start early in the morning and work as long as possible. The decision was also made to eat breakfast and lunch at the training centre. I arrived the first morning thinking surely there would be something there I could eat. WRONG. What they considered breakfast consisted of GIANT muffins and croissants, tea and coffee—there weren't even any jugs of water. Lunch was a huge tray of sandwiches (all on white buns or croissants) and a few carrot sticks. There was a big salad with the dressing already tossed in. Although it was some kind of oil and vinegar dressing, it was sooo sweet. We were on our own for dinner.

"I decided I needed to take control over the meals I could. When I returned to the hotel, I requested that a small fridge be delivered to my room. I then went to the grocery store, where I bought Fibre 1 cereal, skim milk, fruit and disposable bowls, cutlery and bottled water. The next morning I had my breakfast before heading out and felt so much better for it.

"When I arrived at the training centre, I spoke with the girl responsible for organizing and asked her to direct me to the person preparing our lunches. I spoke to the nicest "little" lady from the cafeteria and explained that I can't eat sandwiches laden with butter and mayonnaise, and that I needed a salad not all dressed. She was more than happy to oblige. That afternoon, along with all the sandwiches was a plate of cold meat (not non-fat but okay), cut-up veggies, half a boiled egg and a big pickle. There was salad with nothing on it and a small container of oil and vinegar with no sugar added. I was happy.

"I will admit that I did have a cocktail after work when everyone met before dinner, but I limited myself to one. I know first-hand that alcohol dismisses willpower. I ate dinner out with the group but was as careful as I could be. This allowed me to go to bed without feeling guilty over what I ate that day. I did this for the rest of my stay.

"Overall, I know there were things I ate that weren't green-light, but I feel really good about how I handled things. Prior to this, I would never have said a word and just ate what was provided for me just so I wouldn't bring attention to myself. But now I realize I am the only one who can control what I eat; I am responsible for myself. I wasn't the least bit embarrassed, and no one said a word about my special requests. It was really no big deal, after all. Best of all, I feel in control and that feels so good." —Beverley

Wow, that's tremendous, Beverley! Good luck, everyone, taking control of your meals while away from home!

Week 5 Weight: _____

Week 5 Waist: _____

Week 5 Hips: _____

Week 5 Diary

_____

_____

_____

_____

_____

_____

_____

_____

_____

_____

_____

_____

_____

_____

_____

_____

_____

Week 5 Optional Meal Plan

	BREAKFAST	SNACK	LUNCH	SNACK	DINNER	SNACK
MON	Homey Oatmeal (p. 204) with chopped apple	Cranberry Cinnamon Bran Muffin (p. 271)	Open-face chicken sandwich with lettuce, tomato and onion and Basic G.I. Salad (p. 221)	Laughing Cow Light cheese with crispbread	Easy-Bake Lasagna (p. 237) and Caesar Salad (p. 222)	Mixed berries tossed in lime juice with sour cream
TUES	Mini Breakfast Puffs (p. 208)	Fruit yogurt	G.I. Pasta Salad (p. 225)	Hummus with carrot and celery sticks	G.I. Fish Fillet (p. 244) asparagus, carrots and new potatoes	Orange and almonds
WED	Homemade Muesli (p. 205) with skim milk and fruit yogurt	Cranberry Cinnamon Bran Muffin (p. 271)	1/2 whole wheat pita with canned light tuna, lettuce, tomato and cucumber, and Basic G.I. Salad (p. 221)	Babybel Gouda Lite cheese with crispbread	Chicken Curry (p. 252) and Raita Salad (p. 219)	Apple Pie Cookie (p. 282) and glass of skim milk
THURS	Homey Oatmeal (p. 204) with blueberries	Small apple and glass of skim milk	Quick and Easy Chicken Noodle Soup (p. 216) and Basic G.I Salad (p. 221)	Crunchy Chickpeas (p. 270)	Vegetable Crumble (p. 233) and Tabbouleh Salad (p. 226)	1/2 nutrition bar
FRI	All-Bran Buds with skim milk, peach slices and sliced almonds	Fruit yogurt	Mixed Bean Salad (p. 227)	Laughing Cow Light cheese with crispbread	Chicken Fried Rice (p. 251)	Mixed berries tossed in lime juice with sour cream
SAT	Western Omelette (p. 212)	1/2 nutrition bar	Greek Salad (p. 223)	Hummus with carrot and celery sticks	Beef and Eggplant Chili (p. 263) and Basic G.I. Salad (p. 221)	Apple Pie Cookie (p. 282) and glass of skim milk
SUN	Oatmeal Buttermilk Pancakes (p. 207) with strawberries	Orange and almonds	Tuscan White Bean Soup, (p. 215) and Basic G.I. Salad (p. 221)	Babybel Gouda Lite cheese with crispbread	Pork Medallions Dijon (p. 266), green beans, carrots and new potatoes	Piece of Plum Crumble (p. 278)

Week 5 Grocery List for Meal Plan

PRODUCE
Almonds (whole and sliced)
Apples
Asparagus
Baby spinach
Bean sprouts
Bell peppers (red and green)
Blueberries (fresh or frozen)
Broccoli
Carrots
Celery
Cranberries (dried)
Cucumbers (English and field)
Eggplant
Fresh herbs (chives, mint, flat-leaf parsley,
   sage, tarragon, thyme)
Garlic
Green beans
Green onions
Kale
Leeks
Lemons
Lettuce (iceberg, leaf and Romaine)
Mixed nuts
Mushrooms
Onions (yellow and red)
Oranges
Peaches (fresh or canned in juice or water)
Potatoes (new, small)
Prune plums (e.g., damson or Italian)
Raisins
Sesame seeds
Strawberries
Sunflower seeds, shelled and unsalted
Sweet potato
Tofu (firm)
Tomatoes (plum)
Zucchini

DELI
Feta cheese (light)
Hummus (light)
Kalamata olives
Parmesan cheese, grated

BAKERY
100% stone-ground whole wheat bread
Crispbread (e.g., Wasa Fibre)
Whole wheat pita bread

FISH COUNTER
Fish fillets (salmon or trout)

MEAT COUNTER
Back bacon
Chicken breasts (boneless, skinless)
Ground beef (extra-lean)
Pork tenderloins

BEANS (LEGUMES) AND CANNED VEGETABLES
Chickpeas
Kidney beans (red and white)
Mixed beans
Diced tomatoes
Plum tomatoes
Tomato paste

PASTA AND SAUCES
Lasagna (whole wheat)
Rotini or penne (whole wheat)
Small pasta (e.g., ditali or tubetti)
Light tomato sauce (no added sugar)
Low-fat pasta sauce

SOUP AND CANNED SEAFOOD AND MEAT
Anchovy fillets
Chicken stock (low-fat, low-sodium)

Tuna (light, in water)
Vegetable stock (low-fat, low-sodium)

GRAINS AND SIDE DISHES
Basmati rice
Brown rice
Bulgur
Flaxseeds

INTERNATIONAL FOODS
Sesame oil
Soy sauce (low-sodium)
Tahini

COOKING OIL, VINEGAR, SALAD DRESSINGS AND PICKLES
Dijon mustard
Mayonnaise (fat-free)
Oil (canola and extra-virgin olive)
Red wine vinegar
Vegetable cooking oil spray (canola or olive oil)
Worcestershire sauce

SNACKS
Applesauce (unsweetened)
Nutrition bars (e.g., ZonePerfect, Balance Bar)

BAKING
Baking powder
Baking soda
Cornstarch
Oat bran
Spices (ground cardamom, cayenne pepper, chili powder, ground cinnamon, ground cumin, curry powder, ground ginger, ground nutmeg, dried oregano, black pepper, red pepper flakes, salt, dried thyme)
Splenda
Vanilla

Wheat bran
Wheat germ
Whole wheat flour

BREAKFAST FOODS
All-Bran Buds cereal
Oatmeal (large-flake oats)

BEVERAGES
White wine

DAIRY CASE
Babybel Gouda Lite cheese
Buttermilk
Cheddar cheese (low-fat)
Cottage cheese (1%)
Fruit yogurt (non-fat with sweetener)
Laughing Cow Light cheese
Liquid eggs (e.g., Naturegg Break Free)
Milk (skim)
Mozzarella cheese (part-skim)
Plain yogurt (non-fat)
Soft margarine (non-hydrogenated, light)
Sour cream (low-fat)
Whole omega-3 eggs

FROZEN FOODS
Mixed berries
Peas (or fresh)

Week 6

Unrealistic Expectations

This week I want to address the critical issue of unrealistic expectations. Unfortunately, in this instant-gratification society, we tend to want immediate results. Even though it took us years to gain the weight we currently have, we expect to lose it extremely quickly. But you can't address a long-term problem like being overweight with a short-term solution. Going to extremes by skipping snacks and cutting calories to a dangerously low level just won't work. Slow, steady weight loss is the only healthy and clinically proven way to lose weight permanently. This is why you need a weight-loss plan you can live with for the long haul, which is what the G.I. Diet is all about. One pound a week is the average that most people lose, and it is certainly nothing to sniff at—have you ever seen a pound of fat? It's a substantial amount! And yet look at some of the comments I received from e-Clinic participants:

> "Disappointed with my week of 'progress.' I stuck to the program pretty good, I even cut back on bread when I wasn't losing at the first of the week. Still only lost one pound." —Diane

> "Feeling disappointed at the small weight loss this week and the little or no change in measurements. I have gone over my meals for the past week to see if there is something I might have done better." —Kathy, who lost two pounds in one week

> "Small weight loss . . . I'll need to get some exercise to start burning off more weight."
> —Ross, who lost three pounds in one week

> "Thought maybe I would have lost a little more weight, but patience has never been a virtue for me . . ." —another Kathy, who lost four pounds in one week

All of these people should be feeling happy about their weight loss and proud of their achievements. How unfortunate that they can't give themselves the pat on the back that they so well deserve! Impatience and disappointment with weight-loss success is dangerous: it can derail you from the healthy track you're on and make you want to give up. Just read the following letter from Pat:

> "I am really disappointed with myself, as I have only lost one pound this week. I really want the weight to come off faster than it is . . . I have to tell you, this past Wednesday, mid-afternoon, I started thinking that I was going to pack this program in. I was thinking again about how the weight wasn't coming off fast enough. But I stopped myself, and asked myself, what really is going on here? Was I hungry, tired or thirsty? I came to the revelation that I was tired and really thirsty. Once I stopped and took a rest and had something to drink, I got refocused. I knew in my heart that quitting wasn't what I wanted to do."

People often fail on diets because they have unrealistic weight-loss expectations and become impatient. It's great that Pat was able to refocus and stick with the program. She had been losing an average of over one pound per week, and at that rate she would be reaching her target weight in only nine months. In less than a year she could be at her ideal weight, wearing the clothes she wanted and enjoying her renewed energy and improved health! When you consider the number of years it took to put on the weight, nine months is certainly not an unreasonable timeframe. You know that you are eating in a healthy and nutritious way that is benefiting your body while you reduce. One pound per week is right on target. Yes, there are instances where people have lost three to four pounds per week, but they then frequently hit a plateau and their weight loss averages out to a more normal level. It all depends upon your metabolism, the amount of weight you have to lose, and the degree to which you stick to the green-light way of eating.

Here's what can happen if you lose too much too fast:

> "This last week I am very impressed with my weight loss, but I have been feeling really foggy. I have vertigo and it has been a very bad week for it. I had to leave work early on Friday due to dizziness. I still feel really foggy today. Do you think that it is due to the diet?" —Tammy

Tammy had been losing an average of three pounds per week for six weeks, and I was concerned that she was overdoing things. I suggested she check that her portion sizes were in line with my recommendations and that she was eating her regular three meals and three snacks per day. I also asked her to see her doctor in case there was some other health issue that needed to be addressed.

To end on a positive note, here's a note I received from Jenny:

> "One pound a week for me is really good compared to what I was doing on Weight Watchers (which was about 0.2 pounds a week—very frustrating!)."

Week 6 Weight:_____

Week 6 Waist:_____

Week 6 Hips:_____

Week 6 Diary

_____

_____

_____

_____

_____

_____

_____

Week 6 Optional Meal Plan

	BREAKFAST	SNACK	LUNCH	SNACK	DINNER	SNACK
MON	Homey Oatmeal (p. 204) with chopped apple	Carrot Muffin (p. 272)	Open-face lean deli ham sandwich with lettuce, tomato, red pepper and grainy mustard, and Basic G.I. Salad (p. 221)	Laughing Cow Light cheese with crispbread	Fettuccine Primavera (p. 231), and Caesar Salad (p. 222)	Mixed berries tossed in lime juice with sour cream
TUES	Mini Breakfast Puffs (p. 208)	Fruit yogurt	Waldorf Chicken and Rice Salad (p. 228)	Hummus with carrot and celery sticks	Ginger Wasabi Halibut (p. 246), Cold Noodle Salad with Cucumber and Sesame (p. 224), snow peas and carrots	Orange and almonds
WED	Homemade Muesli (p. 205) with skim milk and fruit yogurt	Carrot Muffin (p. 272)	Cottage cheese with apple and grapes, and Basic G.I. Salad (p. 221)	Babybel Gouda Lite cheese with crispbread	Chicken Tarragon with Mushrooms (p. 256) broccoli, and basmati rice	Pecan Brownie (p. 283) and glass of skim milk
THURS	Homey Oatmeal (p. 204) with blueberries	Small apple and glass of skim milk	Minestrone Soup, (p. 214) and Basic G.I. Salad (p. 221)	Crunchy Chickpeas (p. 270)	Meatloaf (p. 261), green beans, carrots and new potatoes	1/2 nutrition bar
FRI	All-Bran Buds with skim milk, peach slices, and sliced almonds	Fruit yogurt	1/2 whole wheat pita with deli turkey, lettuce, tomato and cucumber, and Basic G.I. Salad (p. 221)	Laughing Cow Light cheese with crispbread	Bean and Onion Pizza (p. 235)	Mixed berries tossed in lime juice with sour cream
SAT	Italian Omelette (p. 210)	1/2 nutrition bar	Crab Salad in Tomato Shells (p. 229)	Hummus with carrot and celery sticks	Grilled Tuna with Chimichurri Sauce (p. 247) asparagus, and new potatoes	Pecan Brownie (p. 283) and glass of skim milk
SUN	Cinnamon French Toast (p. 206) with back bacon	Orange and almonds	Ham and Lentil Soup (p. 217) and Basic G.I. Salad (p. 221)	Babybel Gouda Lite cheese with crispbread	Orange Chicken with Almonds (p. 255), green beans, and basmati rice	Slice of Apple Raspberry Coffee Cake (p. 279)

Week 6 Grocery List for Meal Plan

PRODUCE
Almonds (whole and sliced)
Apples
Asparagus
Baby spinach
Bell peppers (red and green)
Blueberries (fresh or frozen)
Broccoli
Carrots
Celery
Cucumbers (English and field)
Fresh herbs (basil, chives, cilantro, flat-leaf
   parsley)
Garlic
Ginger root
Grapes
Green beans
Green onions
Lemon
Lettuce (leaf and Romaine)
Limes
Mushrooms
Onions (yellow and red)
Oranges
Peaches (fresh or canned in juice or water)
Pecans
Potatoes (new, small)
Raisins
Raspberries
Sesame seeds
Snow peas
Strawberries
Sun-dried tomatoes
Sunflower seeds, shelled and unsalted
Tofu (firm)
Tomatoes (large beefsteak and plum)
Walnuts
Zucchini (yellow)

DELI
Feta cheese (low-fat)
Hummus
Lean deli ham
Lean deli turkey
Parmesan cheese, grated

BAKERY
100% stone-ground whole wheat bread
Crispbread (e.g., Wasa Fibre)
Whole wheat pita bread

FISH COUNTER
Frozen crab
Halibut fillets
Tuna steaks ($1/2$-inch thick)

MEAT COUNTER
Back bacon
Chicken breasts (boneless, skinless)
Ground beef (extra-lean)

BEANS (LEGUMES) AND
CANNED VEGETABLES
Chickpeas
Kidney beans (red and white)
Lentils
Plum tomatoes
Tomato purée

PASTA AND SAUCES
Capellini or spaghettini (whole wheat)
Fettuccini or linguine (whole wheat)
low-fat pasta sauce
Small pasta (e.g., ditali or tubetti)

SOUP AND CANNED SEAFOOD AND MEAT
Anchovy fillets
Chicken stock (low-fat, low-sodium)
Vegetable stock (low-fat, low-sodium)
GRAINS AND SIDE DISHES
Basmati rice
Flaxseeds

INTERNATIONAL FOODS
Mirin (or sweet sherry)
Rice vinegar
Soy sauce (low-sodium)
Sesame seeds (toasted)
Tahini
Wasabi powder

COOKING OIL, VINEGAR, SALAD DRESSINGS AND PICKLES
Buttermilk salad dressing (low-fat, low-sugar)
Dijon mustard
Grainy mustard
Oil (canola and extra-virgin olive)
Vegetable cooking oil spray (canola or olive oil)
Red wine vinegar
Worcestershire sauce

SNACKS
Nutrition bars (e.g., ZonePerfect, Balance Bar)

BAKING
Active dry yeast
Baking powder
Baking soda
Brown sugar substitute
Cornstarch
Oat bran
Spices (cayenne pepper, ground cinnamon, ground ginger, ground nutmeg, dried

oregano, black pepper, red pepper flakes, salt, dried tarragon, dried thyme)
Splenda
Unsweetened cocoa powder
Vanilla
Wheat bran
Wheat germ
Whole wheat flour

BREAKFAST FOODS
All-Bran Buds cereal
Oatmeal (large-flake oats)

BEVERAGES
Tomato juice
Vegetable cocktail juice
Vermouth or white wine

DAIRY CASE
Babybel Gouda Lite cheese
Buttermilk
Fruit yogurt (non-fat with sweetener)
Laughing Cow Light cheese
Liquid eggs (e.g., Naturegg, Break Free)
Milk (skim)
Mozzarella cheese (part-skim)
Soft margarine (non-hydrogenated, light)
Sour cream (low-fat)
Whole omega-3 eggs

FROZEN FOODS
Peas (or fresh)
Mixed berries

Week 7

Emotional Eating

This week we cover the question of emotional eating, frequently described as "using food for comfort." I have asked my wife, Dr. Ruth Gallop, who is Professor Emeritus at the University of Toronto, to write this section, as one of her specialties is childhood trauma and how that plays out in adult life. This has given her considerable insight into the role food plays in helping people deal with their emotional issues. We realize that this is a very large topic but hope to provide you with some guidance. Here are her thoughts.

We all eat for comfort to a lesser or greater extent. When we are sick, many of us have favourite foods—often foods from our childhood that we associate with being looked after. There are foods we eat rarely and foods we could eat every day—often foods that make us feel good or satiated.

When we have reasonably balanced lives, food plays an important but not dominant role in our day-to-day lives. When our lives are out of balance and we don't feel good about certain aspects of our lives, food can take over. When we don't feel good about ourselves, food can be a powerful and damaging force. This is particularly true for women, because our society is fixated on how we should look. Putting aside all the health reasons for being at a "normal" weight, our society just doesn't approve of fat people. And more importantly, fat people often don't approve of themselves.

Eating to feel better is usually preceded by negative feelings. For some people these feelings may include sadness, loneliness or even a sense of boredom. For others the feelings can be more in the range of anger, irritability or high stress. These feelings can lead to a vicious eating cycle that it goes something like this:

> I feel angry/bored/sad/bad about myself (low self-esteem) → so I eat
> to feel better → I experience a brief blood sugar high and feel better
> → I experience a blood sugar crash and feel terrible → I feel bad
> about myself for eating, for failing → so I eat to feel better . . . and
> around I go.

In many situations the original reasons for feeling bad about oneself or getting angry, overwhelmed or disappointed may have origins in childhood, but

overeating, negative body image and low self-esteem are the present conse-
quence. We do not usually make a conscious link between past events and current behaviour. For example, when we were children, parental approval and love
may have been connected with food via treats or eating all that was put in front
of us. Or we may have been punished (love withdrawn) if we didn't eat our vegetables. Eating becomes connected with trying to recapture that good feeling of
being loved. Although we are unaware of these motives or psychological reasons
for the behaviour, we have done it for so long it becomes part of our food and eating habits.

Rick's mother cannot bear to see food left unfinished on the plate, regardless
of whether a person is still hungry. At ninety-seven years of age, she still says, "I
do like to see a clean plate," when all the food on the table has disappeared. I
have learned to deal with this learned behaviour—a behaviour that earned Rick
love and approval from his mother when he was a child—by never putting excess
food on the table at mealtimes or putting out bowls of food for individual selection. Otherwise, Rick's impulse will be to finish the food, and he will unconsciously graze.

How do you change eating behaviours that you learned as a child? First, you
have taken the most important step by removing all red-light food from the
house and making a conscious decision to eat only green-light foods—a huge
step! Make sure you reward yourself for this accomplishment. Give yourself a
treat (just make sure it isn't a red-light food)!

Become conscious of your eating habits. For example, when you walk in the
front door, is your first stop the fridge or snack cupboard? When you have had a
bad day at work or the kids have been a hassle, do you deal with it by eating
something sweet or high-fat? When you feel bored and have nothing structured
to do, is food the first thing you think of? Are you unable to watch TV without
snacking, so large amounts of food pass into your mouth without you realizing?
I have one piece of dark chocolate most evenings if I am watching TV. The other
night I realized I was in the middle of eating a second piece with no memory of
reaching down and picking it up!

Take a day or two to jot down your eating patterns, noting when automatic
behaviours take over and when it is most difficult for you to avoid eating in

excess. You'll soon begin to recognize your "at-risk" situations. If food comforts you when you're stressed or setting unrealistic expectations for yourself, such as getting all the errands done, cooking all the meals and doing all the child care, you'll start to recognize your patterns and can then consider alternative ways to cope, for example, sharing tasks with others.

Some emotional eating habits to watch out for include:

- **Grazing.** This is a well-established teenage habit that many have not grown out of. If you cannot pass a fridge without opening it, grazing is a habit for you.
- **Eating when stressed, angry, irritable, tired or frustrated.**
- **Eating when sad, bored or lonely.**
- **Eating too quickly.** Never gobble your food. Remember, it takes twenty to thirty minutes for the stomach to tell the brain it is full.
- **Eating unconsciously.** Never eat from large packages of food. Instead, put the small portion you plan to eat in a bowl or on a plate.
- **Eating too-large portions**. Thanks to fast-food and family restaurants, many portion sizes have doubled in recent years, and we have brought this "portion distortion" into our homes.
- **Always eating during any social activity**, such as sports events, visits and having coffee with a friend.

Once you have recognized your own unhealthy eating behaviours, change by modifying one behaviour at a time. For example, if you usually walk in the front door and immediately go to the fridge to get a snack, consider it one of your snack times and ensure that you have a green-light snack ready. If you usually eat while watching television in the evenings, make a list of pleasurable activities you could be doing instead of eating. How about putting together a photo album, knitting or even ironing while watching your favourite shows? Or are there pleasurable things you could do instead of watching TV, like doing a crossword puzzle, going for a walk, taking a class to learn a fun hobby or even having a hot bath? Substituting pleasurable activities helps break the vicious cycle I have described above. To start the process, write out a list of substitute activities you enjoy.

Substitute Activities List

1. _____

2. _____

3. _____

4. _____

5. _____

6. _____

This list will be an important tool to help break those bad eating habits. Use it until you feel sure that your new behaviours and eating patterns are your new habits. And don't beat yourself up if you slip—it happens to all of us. Just get back on the wagon. Having the determination to do this program deserves a pat on the back, so be sure to reward yourself for your small triumphs—go to a show or game, or buy some flowers or a new CD.

Emotional eating is a subject that resonated with e-Clinic participants, many of whom have struggled with their weight since childhood.

"I had some emotional eating this week. On Tuesday, my doctor told me my x-rays were clear for pneumonia, but there were spots in the lower lungs. That night I had a steak and some red wine. I figured if I had lung cancer I'd lose weight anyway, so what the hell? Had a CT scan on Wednesday and on Friday found out the spots were scars from previous bouts of bronchitis/pneumonia. That led to a celebratory glass of wine (or two) with dinner. I'm back on track now, but this has been a roller coaster week." —Karen

"I do recognize that for the past four years as a single parent I have often chosen to eat without any sensation of hunger in an effort to deal with (maybe avoid dealing with) being on my own, the isolation of

single parenting and my disappointment in myself for being in this situation, or just generally feeling sorry for myself at times and not wanting to deny myself a 'treat.' I do recognize that the emotional aspect of my situation has only been made worse by my feelings of upset with myself for being so heavy, and that I have to work hard to reward and console myself in different ways, to build in treats that are not edible."
—Bernadette

"I have gained two pounds this week. Disappointed and angry with myself definitely. I can only say that this is a result of emotional eating this week. My stress level at work was at a high level . . . One day mid-week, my commuting friend bought me a large chocolate-covered marshmallow on a stick, as she knew that this was a treat my mother and I shared at this time of the year. In addition to this, I have been having a lot of dreams of my deceased parents . . . All I can say is, 'lesson learned,' and now another week begins and I must get back on track because losing the weight is extremely important to me . . . I didn't realize until I started this program how much of an emotional eater I am." —Pat

"Your wife's comments on the emotional aspect of eating and food really hit home. I have to constantly work on this. I think we all know we are doing it, but at the time you do it anyway and fuel the cycle. I'm looking at some sort of hobby to turn to instead of the fridge. Or I guess I could take up smoking and drinking instead . . . Just kidding!" —Ross

"I've been through a lot in the past few years (a divorce followed by an abusive relationship), and I know I gained all the extra weight in some effort to 'protect' myself. I am trying to learn to love myself in ways that do not involve reaching for food as a means of consoling myself. I have a long way to go, but I have the basic tools—plus, I'm on my own now and SAFE. The stronger I get financially and emotionally, the more I care about my health and appearance." —Nancy

Keep in mind that as you lose weight you will feel better not only physically but also psychologically. Being successful will improve your self-esteem. Feeling better about how you look is the best reinforcement for holding back on red-light foods and breaking those bad eating habits. You will notice your body changing, and others will too. As you start to experience success in permanent weight reduction, you will think of yourself as successful. Successful people hold their bodies differently and interact with people differently. As a reader once said, "I no longer hide behind a tree every time a camera comes out." You may find you feel safe enough to come out into the world. Let people compliment you.

Week 7 Weight: _____

Week 7 Waist: _____

Week 7 Hips: _____

Week 7 Diary

_____

_____

_____

_____

_____

_____

_____

_____

Week 7 Optional Meal Plan

	BREAKFAST	SNACK	LUNCH	SNACK	DINNER	SNACK
MON	Homey Oatmeal (p. 204) with chopped apple	Apple Bran Muffin (p. 273)	Open-face chicken sandwich with lettuce, tomato and onion, and Basic G.I. Salad (p. 221)	Laughing Cow Light cheese with crispbread	Rigatoni with Mini Meatballs (p. 264) and Caesar Salad (p. 222)	Mixed berries tossed in lime juice with sour cream
TUES	Mini Breakfast Puffs (p. 208)	Fruit yogurt	G.I. Pasta Salad (p. 225)	Hummus with carrot and celery sticks	Citrus-Poached Haddock (p. 245), green beans and new potatoes	Orange and almonds
WED	Homemade Muesli (p. 205) with skim milk and fruit yogurt	Apple Bran Muffin (p. 273)	1/2 whole wheat pita with canned light tuna, lettuce, tomato and cucumber, and Basic G.I. Salad (p. 221)	Babybel Gouda Lite cheese with crispbread	Chicken Jambalaya (p. 254) and broccoli	Creamy Lemon Square (p. 284) and glass of skim milk
THURS	Homey Oatmeal (p. 204) with blueberries	Small apple and glass of skim milk	Quick and Easy Chicken Noodle Soup (p. 216) and Basic G.I. Salad (p. 221)	Crunchy Chickpeas (p. 270)	Barley Risotto with Leeks, Lemon and Peas (p. 232), and Tabbouleh Salad (p. 226)	1/2 nutrition bar
FRI	All-Bran Buds with skim milk, peach slices and sliced almonds	Fruit yogurt	Mixed Bean Salad (p. 227)	Laughing Cow Light cheese with crispbread	Thai Red Curry Shrimp Pasta (p. 243)	Mixed berries tossed in lime juice with sour cream
SAT	Vegetarian Omelette (p. 211)	1/2 nutrition bar	Greek Salad (p. 223)	Hummus with carrot and celery sticks	Zesty Barbecued Chicken, (p. 258), Tangy Red and Green Coleslaw (p. 220), and new potatoes	Creamy Lemon Square (p. 284) and glass of skim milk
SUN	Oatmeal Buttermilk Pancakes (p. 207) with strawberries	Orange and almonds	Tuscan White Bean Soup (p. 215), and Basic G.I. Salad (p. 221)	Babybel Gouda Lite cheese with crispbread	Pork Tenderloin with Apple Compote (p. 268), Brussels sprouts, carrots and new potatoes	Piece of Berry Crumble (p. 277)

Week 7 Grocery List for Meal Plan

PRODUCE
Almonds (whole and sliced)
Apples
Bell peppers (red and green)
Blueberries (fresh or frozen)
Broccoli
Brussels sprouts
Cabbage (green and red)
Carrots
Celery
Cucumbers
Currants
Eggplant
Fresh herbs (chives, cilantro, flat-leaf parsley,
  mint, rosemary, sage and thyme)
Garlic
Green beans
Green onions
Kale
Leek
Lemons
Lettuce (leaf, iceberg and Romaine)
Limes
Mushrooms
Onions (yellow and red)
Oranges
Peaches (fresh or canned in juice or water)
Pecans
Potatoes (new, small)
Strawberries
Sunflower seeds, shelled and unsalted
Tomatoes (plum)
Zucchini

DELI
Feta cheese (light)
Hummus (light)

Kalamata olives
Parmesan cheese, grated

BAKERY
100% stone-ground whole wheat bread
Crispbread (e.g., Wasa Fibre)
Whole wheat pita bread

FISH COUNTER
Haddock fillets
Shrimp (large raw)

MEAT COUNTER
Chicken breasts (boneless, skinless)
Lean ground chicken or turkey
Pork tenderloin

BEANS (LEGUMES) AND CANNED VEGETABLES
Chickpeas
Kidney beans (red and white)
Mixed beans
Plum tomatoes
Stewed tomatoes
Tomato paste

PASTA AND SAUCES
Rotini or penne (whole wheat)
Marcaroni or small shells (whole wheat)
Rigatoni (whole wheat)
Spagettini or linguine (whole wheat)
Small pasta (e.g., ditali or tubetti)
Light tomato sauce

SOUP AND CANNED SEAFOOD AND MEAT
Anchovy fillets
Chicken stock (low-fat, low-sodium)
Tuna (light, in water)
Vegetable stock (low-fat, low-sodium)

GRAINS AND SIDE DISHES
Barley
Brown rice
Bulgur
Flaxseeds

INTERNATIONAL FOODS
Tahini
Thai red curry paste

COOKING OIL, VINEGAR, SALAD DRESSINGS AND PICKLES
Cider vinegar
Dijon mustard
Mayonnaise (fat-free)
Oil (canola and extra-virgin olive)
Red wine vinegar
Vegetable cooking oil spray (canola or olive oil)
Worcestershire sauce

SNACKS
Applesauce (unsweetened)
Nutrition bars (e.g., ZonePerfect, Balance Bar)

BAKING
Baking powder
Baking soda
Brown sugar substitute
Cornstarch
Ground almonds
Oat bran
Spices (ground allspice, bay leaves, cayenne pepper, celery seeds, chili powder, ground cinnamon, ground cloves, ground cumin, dried oregano, black pepper, dried sage, salt, dried thyme)
Splenda
Vanilla
Wheat bran

Wheat germ
Whole wheat flour

BREAKFAST FOODS
All-Bran Buds cereal
Oatmeal (large-flake oats)

BEVERAGES
Apple juice (unsweetened)
Dry white wine (or vermouth)

DAIRY CASE
Babybel Gouda Lite cheese
Buttermilk
Cheddar cheese (low-fat)
Fruit yogurt (non-fat with sweetener)
Laughing Cow Light cheese
Liquid eggs (e.g., Naturegg, Break Free)
Milk (skim)
Orange juice (unsweetened)
Soft margarine (non-hydrogenated, light)
Sour cream (low-fat)
Whole omega-3 eggs

FROZEN FOODS
Frozen apple juice concentrate
Mixed berries
Peas (or fresh)

Week 8

Reaching a Plateau

When you're rigorously adhering to the green-light way and have been steadily losing weight for many successive weeks, it's difficult to accept that the weight loss should suddenly stall. Unfair as it may be, it is inevitable. Weight loss never occurs in a straight line, but always in a series of steps or plateaus, as all of our e-Clinic participants discovered at one point or another:

"I am totally surprised and very disappointed. This week I made sure that I ate only green, knowing that I had two dinners out for my birthday. I even went online and checked the menus at both places so I could go in knowing exactly what I was going to have and not be tempted by everything else. I skipped the bread basket, the desserts, had grilled chicken and salad with vinaigrette dressing at one place, and grilled salmon, fresh beans and baby carrots, and salad with vinaigrette dressing on my birthday. The only thing I did have was a small glass of wine. No cake, didn't eat one of my favourite cookies fresh from Tim Hortons that were bought by one of the girls I ride in with on the bus, since we couldn't have a cake, she said. I was so pleased with myself—that was until I stepped on the scale this morning and it showed the 1.5 pound GAIN and no change in measurements. I just don't understand. I'm at a loss, frustrated and very disappointed." —Kathy

"Battling a tough weekly result. I'm a little baffled at my lack of weight loss this week, and due to the results I had a bout of emotional eating with a box of Timbits. I find it really frustrating (and I've been here before) to do a total 180 on my eating and not have any weight come off." —Sandra

"Well, I have found a plateau, but since I knew it was out there waiting for me and this is a marathon not a sprint, I'm okay with it—after a few moments of 'black cloud.' As long as things keep moving forward . . ." —Ross

Many factors show up on the scale: stress, water retention, hormonal shifts, change in exercise schedules, even seasonality. The body tends to naturally want to put on weight for winter and lose a bit for summer due to the feast-and-famine cycles from deep in our ancestral past. Estrogen levels in particular can influence how much water you retain, which is why women experience sudden short-term changes in weight, especially before a period—and even more so during menopause. Menopause, which can go on for up to ten years, can impact a woman's weight in two ways. First, estrogen levels decrease, causing erratic swings in water retention and blood sugar levels. When your blood sugar levels drop, your brain calls for more sugar, making you want to reach out for those red-light foods, which will temporarily give you a boost and make you feel better in the short term. However, the sugar high will cause your insulin to kick in, quickly bringing your blood sugar levels down to another low. We know all about this relentless cycle. That's why it's so important to eat only green-light foods, because they will help stabilize your blood sugar and mood.

Second, menopause will slow your metabolic rate, or the rate at which your body burns calories. As you're aware, to lose weight, you have to use up more calories than your body takes in. So if you are burning fewer calories, your rate of weight loss will slow. This is why it can be more of a challenge to lose weight during menopause.

So for many reasons, your weight can fluctuate significantly even day to day. This is why I suggest you restrict your weigh-in to once a week, and why I think it would be better to weigh in only once a month. Then you'd avoid the disappointment of these short-term aberrations and focus on your long-term success.

You are playing the averages and must have patience. Just keep on the green-light track and the weight will continue to come off. Some e-Clinic participants also wondered why they sometimes seemed to be losing inches but not pounds, and sometimes pounds but not inches. Remember, everyone is different, and weight loss doesn't ever happen in a straight line; eventually both the inches and pounds will come off—guaranteed!

So don't let an irregularity on the scale get you down. Though nothing is quite as frustrating as hitting a weight-loss plateau, if you hang in there—and don't use food to console yourself—you will reach your weight-loss target. Here is how some e-Clinic participants tried to focus on the positive as they came to terms with their plateaus:

> "I thought I had done well this week and was sure I had a good loss . . . It was disappointing when the scale said I'd lost only half a pound and virtually nothing in inches. I can't believe that with the amount of weight I have to lose my body would be considering plateauing yet! I know I feel good and that I made good decisions this week, but I just didn't see any rewards. I don't know how much my monthly cycle plays in this, as I was on all week . . . Oh well, as they say, Rome wasn't built in a day, and I'm not going to lose all this weight in a day, a month or even a year (sounds daunting!)" —Kathy

> "I like to weigh myself daily because I feel it keeps me on track. It does not discourage me. I have always done it that way. The only exception I make is if I know I had a really bad day then I will wait a day to weigh myself. But I have noticed since my weight has been going down that it will be down for a few days then pop back up to the older weight and then a few days later back down it will go. The encouraging part is that each time it goes up it is not as far as the time before." —Diane

> "No weight loss this week, but my other numbers (measurements) are down . . . At this point I have lost 15 pounds, 4.5 inches from waist and 4.5 inches from hips, and my BMI is down from 38.4 to 36. I know the scale is one measurement to use, but that's only one number. I am also looking at my other numbers, and for me, using these other numbers helps keep me from being disappointed when the scale does not move." —Jenny

Week 8 Weight: _____

Week 8 Waist: _____

Week 8 Hips: _____

Week 8 Diary

_____

_____

_____

_____

_____

_____

_____

_____

_____

_____

_____

_____

_____

_____

_____

_____

_____

_____

_____

Week 8 Optional Meal Plan

BREAKFAST	SNACK	LUNCH	SNACK	DINNER	SNACK
Homey Oatmeal (p. 204) with chopped apple	Whole Wheat Fruit Scone (p. 274)	Open-face lean deli ham sandwich with lettuce, tomato, red pepper and grainy mustard, and Basic G.I. Salad (p. 221)	Laughing Cow cheese with crispbread	Salmon Pasta (p. 242)	Mixed berries tossed in lime juice with sour cream
Mini Breakfast Puffs (p. 208)	Fruit yogurt	Waldorf Chicken and Rice Salad (p. 228)	Hummus with carrot and celery sticks	Pan-Seared White Fish with Mandarin Salsa (p. 248), broccoli and basmati rice	Orange and almonds
Homemade Muesli (p. 205) with skim milk and fruit yogurt	Whole Wheat Fruit Scone (p. 274)	Cottage cheese with apple and grapes, and Basic G.I. Salad (p. 221)	Babybel Gouda Lite cheese with crispbread	Chicken Schnitzel (p. 253), green beans, carrots and new potatoes	Slice of Strawberry Tea Bread (p. 275) and glass of skim milk
Homey Oatmeal (p. 204) with blueberries	Small apple and glass of skim milk	Minestrone Soup (p. 214) and Basic G.I. Salad (p. 221)	Crunchy Chickpeas (p. 270)	Mushroom and Gravy Pork Chops (p. 267), asparagus and basmati rice	1/2 nutrition bar
All-Bran Buds with skim milk, peach slices and sliced almonds	Fruit yogurt	1/2 whole wheat pita with deli turkey, lettuce, tomato and cucumber, and Basic G.I. Salad (p. 221)	Laughing Cow cheese with crispbread	Horseradish Burgers (p. 262), and Tabbouleh Salad (p. 226)	Mixed berries tossed in lime juice with sour cream
Back Bacon Omelette (p. 209)	1/2 nutrition bar	Crab Salad in Tomato Shells (p. 229)	Hummus with carrot and celery sticks	Vegetarian Moussaka (p. 239), and basmati rice	Slice of Strawberry Tea Bread (p. 275) and glass of skim milk
Cinnamon French Toast (p. 206) with back bacon	Orange and almonds	Ham and Lentil Soup (p. 217), and Basic G.I. Salad (p. 224)	Babybel Gouda Lite cheese with crispbread	Spicy Roasted Chicken with Tomatoes and Tarragon (p. 257), green beans, and basmati rice	Slice of One-Bowl Chocolate Cake (p. 281), with berries

Week 8 Grocery List for Meal Plan

PRODUCE
Alfalfa sprouts (optional)
Almonds (whole and sliced)
Apples
Asparagus
Baby spinach
Bell peppers (red and green)
Blueberries (fresh or frozen)
Broccoli
Carrots
Celery
Cucumbers
Dried apricots
Eggplants
Fresh herbs (basil, chives, cilantro, flat-leaf
    parsley, mint, tarragon)
Garlic
Grapes
Green beans
Green onions
Lemons
Lettuce (leaf)
Limes
Mushrooms
Onions (yellow and red)
Oranges
Peaches (fresh or canned in juice or water)
Pecans
Potatoes (new, small)
Strawberries
Sun-dried tomatoes
Sunflower seeds, shelled and unsalted
Tomatoes (large beefsteak, plum, and cherry
    or grape)
Walnuts

DELI
Feta cheese (light)
Hummus (light)
Lean deli ham
Lean deli turkey
Light herb and garlic cream cheese
Parmesan cheese, grated

BAKERY
100% stone-ground whole wheat bread
Crispbread (e.g., Wasa Fibre)
Whole wheat breadcrumbs
Whole wheat hamburger buns
Whole wheat pita bread

FISH COUNTER
Frozen crab
Salmon fillet
White fish fillets

MEAT COUNTER
Back bacon
Boneless pork loin chops
Chicken breasts (boneless, skinless)
Ground beef (extra-lean)

**BEANS (LEGUMES) AND
CANNED VEGETABLES**
Chickpeas
Kidney beans (red)
Lentils
Diced tomatoes
Plum tomatoes
Tomato paste

PASTA AND SAUCES
Macaroni (whole wheat)
Small pasta (e.g., ditali or tubetti)

SOUP AND CANNED SEAFOOD AND MEAT
Chicken stock (low-fat, low-sodium)

GRAINS AND SIDE DISHES
Basmati rice
Bulgur

INTERNATIONAL FOODS
Rice vinegar

COOKING OIL, VINEGAR, SALAD DRESSINGS AND PICKLES
Buttermilk salad dressing (low-fat, low-sugar)
Dijon mustard
Grainy mustard
Horseradish
Mayonnaise (fat-free)
Oil (canola and extra-virgin olive)
Red wine vinegar
Steak sauce
Vegetable cooking oil spray (canola or olive oil)
Worcestershire sauce

SNACKS
Applesauce (unsweetened)
Nutrition bars (e.g., ZonePerfect, Balance Bar)
Canned mandarin oranges (no added sugar)

BAKING
Baking powder
Baking soda
Oat bran
Spices (ground allspice, dried basil, cayenne pepper, ground cinnamon, ground cumin, Italian herb seasoning, nutmeg, dried oregano, black pepper, red pepper flakes, salt, dried thyme)
Splenda
Unsweetened cocoa powder

Vanilla
Wheat bran
Wheat germ
Whole wheat flour

BREAKFAST FOODS
All-Bran Buds cereal
Oatmeal (large-flake oats)

BEVERAGES
Apple juice (unsweetened)
Dry white wine (or vermouth)

DAIRY CASE
1% pressed cottage cheese
Babybel Gouda Lite cheese
Buttermilk
Fruit yogurt (non-fat with sweetener)
Laughing Cow Light cheese (extra-low-fat)
Liquid eggs (e.g., Naturegg, Break Free)
Milk (skim)
Orange juice (unsweetened)
Soft margarine (non-hydrogenated, light)
Sour cream (low-fat)

FROZEN FOODS
Mixed berries
Peas (or fresh)

Week 9

Staying Motivated

We are now nearly two-thirds of the way through the first thirteen weeks of the G.I. Diet—it's a great time to reflect on your progress to date and what still needs to be done to keep your motivation high. Over the past eight weeks, e-Clinic participants have reported a wide range of results. Some have taken to the green-light way of eating like the proverbial duck to water, while others have struggled to make the transition from their red-light habits. Most of the problems participants experienced had nothing to do with the diet, but with stress, emotions, work and home pressures, and non-related health issues. The common thread, however, was that they were all determined to get that weight devil off their backs.

This week, I want to discuss keeping determination strong. You wouldn't be human if you didn't feel your resolve starting to waver from time to time. When it does, there are a number of things you can do to encourage yourself to keep going:

1. Remember your initial reasons.
Reread your reasons for wanting to lose weight on page 58. Remember why it was so important to you to slim down when you started this journey, and why you need to persevere.

2. Use physical reminders of your goal.
Keep a picture of an outfit you're going to buy when you reach your goal, or a photograph of a thinner you where you will see it every day:

> "A picture or two of yourself really helps, I think. Although you know you are overweight, your mental picture of yourself is not of an overweight person. I can only speak for myself here. Once I saw some pictures of how I really looked, how I looked to others, and that was a big help in motivating me." —Ross

> "I am using my beautiful red leather coat to motivate me. Last winter, when I went to put it on, it was about 2 inches too small. I was not able to close the zipper. Now, when I put the coat on, I am able to zip it up. Tight, yes, but I know that I have made progress. What an incredible feeling . . . I am determined to wear the coat this winter."

"I had reached the point where I had to buy clothing in the Big Women's section of a shop. I was determined that that was not going to happen again. I dropped almost 25 pounds, and I know I had reached a comfort level with how my old clothing was fitting. I think to some extent not buying new clothing backfired. With my clothes falling off of me, I no longer felt that strain on my waistband if I overindulged. So, I've done two things: 1. I've gone into the closet and found even smaller clothes than the ones that now fit. I am wearing clothes (not out in public!) that are much too tight. The discomfort is a reminder that I've got a long way to go. And 2. I recently went shopping for new clothes. Instead of trying on and buying size 16 (which I am now down to) I found the prettiest things I could find in 12 and 14 which were not available in my size. I tried them on in the dressing room to get an idea of how much more I have to do before I can just walk into a shop and pick up anything I like." —Karen

3. Keep in mind how far you've come.

Compare yourself now to where you were before you started the diet. How much weight have you lost? How much better do your clothes fit you? How has your energy level and health improved? What can you do now that you couldn't do before? Going back to your old eating habits won't seem so tempting when you think how it will undermine all the good things that weight loss has brought you so far.

"I realized this morning that I am no longer experiencing heartburn at night, which is an added bonus." —Nancy

"I did notice yesterday when I put on a sweatshirt from last year that it was big. What a great feeling. When I was putting away my summer clothes, I said to myself, 'I won't be using these again.' What a motivator." —Pat

"This may sound strange, but I am beginning to notice that everything tastes better, and in turn foods that are very salty are almost unpalatable." —Bernadette

"I've officially broken below 260, something I've never accomplished before on any other diet. I'm so excited!" —J

4. Try the "shopping bag cure."

Often, people don't realize how much weight actually weighs. Sounds crazy, but when people tell me they've lost "only" 20 pounds, I ask them to fill a couple of shopping bags with 20 pounds of books and carry them up and down the stairs a few times. Everyone is always glad to put the bags down and report that they had no idea how heavy 20 pounds really is.

So the next time you're feeling uninspired, fill a shopping bag or two with the amount of books or cans of food that equals how much weight you've lost over the last eight weeks of the program and carry them up and down a flight of stairs three times. You'll be amazed at what you've lost, and you'll be relieved to put the bag down. You couldn't have put that weight down weeks ago, when it was still around your waist, hips and thighs!

Keep the bag intact, and add more books or cans as you continue to lose weight. It's a wonderful motivator.

"Many years ago, I had lost a lot of weight. When I was at a 20-pound loss, a dear skinny friend said to me, "Diana, do you realize you have lost the equivalent of a 20-pound bag of potatoes? Just carry that around for a while to see how much you have lost." I have often thought about that. And yes, I have noticed a big difference in my energy level; going up and down steps is not nearly as hard. My joints do not ache as much and my blood pressure is so much better. And my clothes are also fitting better. So even though I've lost 'only 13 pounds,' I am feeling the effects and do not want to go backwards!" —Diane

"At last, I'm below the dreaded 300—never to be seen again! . . . I didn't think this day would ever arrive. Although 21 pounds doesn't seem like a lot if you look at the whole picture, it was my first target in my journey . . . It's 21 pounds in the right direction, and when I held 21 pounds of kitty litter in the store I realized it's a lot of weight to be carrying every day—no wonder my knees and back hurt!" —Kathy

5. Get support.

Buddy up with friends, a spouse or family members who are trying to lose weight. They will give you a sense of camaraderie and encouragement as you strive for your goal, and you can turn to them for support when you need it.

"The BEST way to stay motivated is to do the program with someone else. My 'G.I. Jane' group has been a fantastic source of inspiration and motivation. When one of us is down, the others pick us up. When we are all down at the same time, we have a group meeting and re-kindle the reasons we are doing all of this." —Lynn

"I would like to suggest to everyone that they need to find a good friend to be accountable to. Someone to share with. That is one good thing I have done differently this time. Usually, I do not mention I am dieting to anyone . . . that way 'when' I fail I don't look like a fool again. This time, I have mentioned it to several people. They are also my inspiration to continue. I know they are watching how I eat and how my clothes fit! I know that I can pick any one of them to be accountable to each week if I feel the need. HOWEVER, I know that the person I need to be account-able to the most is ME! I am the one that will benefit by my sticking to this new eating habit and not anyone else!" —Diane

My friend Kathy is also a part of this program. Part of our weekly chat is to check with one another on our progress and to provide support. We are good at giving each other praise when it is appropriate and providing words of encouragement too. We also discuss our accom-plishments and challenges. It really helps to have a good buddy system. It makes the journey easier." —Pat

"My kids are young but very supportive, as I have told them I am trying to make better food choices so that I will be healthy for a long time. (They have decided that this means I will be able to babysit when I am a grandma to their kids! They are only six and nine!)" —Bernadette

"The holiday barrage of social events starts this coming Friday night, but I think I have that one under control. I had a long conversation with a male friend and told him what I have been doing, which was a surprise in itself, as I don't normally share that kind of information. But he was thrilled and is so supportive—it really felt good. And he will also be at the Friday event." —Kathy

6. The $10 cure

This is a motivator that people often stumble upon by accident. The siren song of a red-light lunch draws them into a fast-food chain, where they order a burger with the works, a large french fries and a shake. Mid-afternoon, they feel lousy and can barely keep their eyes open—they've found out the hard way where straying from the green-light path gets you.

"When you mentioned in your book how horrible you'd feel eating red-light foods after going on this diet, you weren't kidding!" —J

"On the couple days I made poor choices, I definitely noticed a difference in how I felt afterwards: depressed, lethargic and a bit nauseated. That, combined with the minute weight loss has encouraged me that I need to avoid any deviations because they have such a trickle-down effect." —Jenny

"Feeling well is a far better treat than whatever red-light food is on offer." —Bernadette

I call this the $10 cure because it's the food version of what immigrants (like me) used to call the "$1,000 cure." Whenever a new arrival, after a long, cold winter in Canada, started to pine for "the old country," the cure was to get on a plane and go home for a week. All the reasons that originally persuaded the person to emigrate would come crashing back, and the thought of flying back to Canada would begin to look pretty good again.

With food, the cure costs less—say, $10. But this is a motivator of last resort only; I certainly don't want to encourage people to abuse their bodies and feel awful! However, if you've been unceasingly pining for red-light foods, go out for lunch with some friends and order a high-G.I. meal—perhaps a couple of slices of double-cheese pizza, a Coke and a brownie. Your mouth may enjoy it, but I guarantee that a couple hours later you'll be regretting the deviation!

Staying motivated is crucial to successful weight loss. It keeps you focused and on the green-light path, and it will get you through the pitfalls you'll encounter. Be sure to use all six of the above strategies—and you probably have a couple of your own that work well. Next week, we'll be discussing the relationship between weight and health—another highly motivating factor as you slim down to your ideal weight.

Week 9 Weight:_____

Week 9 Waist:_____

Week 9 Hips:_____

Week 9 Diary

_____

_____

_____

_____

Week 9 Optional Meal Plan

	BREAKFAST	SNACK	LUNCH	SNACK	DINNER	SNACK
MON	Homey Oatmeal (p. 204) with chopped apple	Cranberry Cinnamon Bran Muffin (p. 271)	Open-face chicken sandwich with lettuce, tomato and onion and Basic G.I. Salad (p. 221)	Laughing Cow Light cheese with crispbread	Easy-Bake Lasagna (p. 237) and Caesar Salad (p. 222)	Mixed berries tossed in lime juice with sour cream
TUES	Mini Breakfast Puffs (p. 208)	Fruit yogurt	G.I. Pasta Salad (p. 225)	Hummus with carrot and celery sticks	G.I. Fish Fillet (p. 244), asparagus, carrots and new potatoes	Orange and almonds
WED	Homemade Muesli (p. 205) with skim milk and fruit yogurt	Cranberry Cinnamon Bran Muffin (p. 271)	1/2 whole wheat pita with canned light tuna, lettuce, tomato and cucumber, and Basic G.I. Salad (p. 221)	Babybel Gouda Lite cheese with crispbread	Chicken Curry (p. 252), and Raita Salad (p. 219)	Apple Pie Cookie (p. 282), and glass of skim milk
THURS	Homey Oatmeal (p. 204) with blueberries	Small apple and glass of skim milk	Quick and Easy Chicken Noodle Soup (p. 216) and Basic G.I. Salad (p. 221)	Crunchy Chickpeas (p. 270)	Vegetable Crumble (p. 233) and Tabbouleh Salad (p. 226)	1/2 nutrition bar
FRI	All-Bran Buds with skim milk, peach slices and sliced almonds	Fruit yogurt	Mixed Bean Salad (p. 227)	Laughing Cow Light cheese with crispbread	Chicken Fried Rice (p. 251)	Mixed berries tossed in lime juice with sour cream
SAT	Western Omelette (p. 212)	1/2 nutrition bar	Greek Salad (p. 223)	Hummus with carrot and celery sticks	Beef and Eggplant Chili (p. 263) and Basic G.I. Salad (p. 221)	Apple Pie Cookie (p. 282) and glass of skim milk
SUN	Oatmeal Buttermilk Pancakes (p. 207) with strawberries	Orange and almonds	Tuscan White Bean Soup (p. 215) and Basic G.I. Salad (p. 221)	Babybel Gouda Lite cheese with crispbread	Pork Medallions Dijon (p. 266), green beans, carrots and new potatoes	Piece of Plum Crumble (p. 278)

Week 9 Grocery List for Meal Plan

PRODUCE
Almonds (whole and sliced)
Apples
Asparagus
Baby spinach
Bean sprouts
Bell peppers (red and green)
Blueberries (fresh or frozen)
Broccoli
Carrots
Celery
Cranberries (dried)
Cucumbers (English and field)
Eggplant
Fresh herbs (chives, mint, flat-leaf parsley,
    sage, tarragon, thyme)
Garlic
Green beans
Green onions
Kale
Leeks
Lemons
Lettuce (iceberg, leaf and Romaine)
Mixed nuts
Mushrooms
Onions (yellow and red)
Oranges
Peaches (fresh or canned in juice or water)
Potatoes (new, small)
Prune plums (e.g., damson or Italian)
Raisins
Sesame seeds
Strawberries
Sunflower seeds, shelled and unsalted
Sweet potato
Tofu (firm)
Tomatoes (plum)
Zucchini

DELI
Feta cheese (light)
Hummus (light)
Kalamata olives
Parmesan cheese, grated

BAKERY
100% stone-ground whole wheat bread
Crispbread (e.g., Wasa Fibre)
Whole wheat pita bread

FISH COUNTER
Fish fillets (salmon or trout)

MEAT COUNTER
Back bacon
Chicken breasts (boneless, skinless)
Ground beef (extra-lean)
Pork tenderloins

**BEANS (LEGUMES) AND
CANNED VEGETABLES**
Chickpeas
Kidney beans (red and white)
Mixed beans
Diced tomatoes
Plum tomatoes
Tomato paste

PASTA AND SAUCES
Lasagna (whole wheat)
Rotini or penne (whole wheat)
Small pasta (e.g., ditali or tubetti)
Light tomato sauce (no added sugar)
Low-fat pasta sauce

SOUP AND CANNED SEAFOOD AND MEAT
Anchovy fillets
Chicken stock (low-fat, low-sodium)
Tuna (light, in water)
Vegetable stock (low-fat, low-sodium)

GRAINS AND SIDE DISHES
Basmati rice
Brown rice
Bulgur
Flaxseeds

INTERNATIONAL FOODS
Sesame oil
Soy sauce (low-sodium)
Tahini

COOKING OIL, VINEGAR, SALAD DRESSINGS AND PICKLES
Dijon mustard
Mayonnaise (fat-free)
Oil (canola and extra-virgin olive)
Red wine vinegar
Vegetable cooking oil spray (canola or olive oil)
Worcestershire sauce

SNACKS
Applesauce (unsweetened)
Nutrition bars (e.g., ZonePerfect, Balance Bar)

BAKING
Baking powder
Baking soda
Cornstarch
Oat bran
Spices (ground cardamom, cayenne pepper, chili powder, ground cinnamon, ground cumin, curry powder, ground ginger, ground nutmeg, dried oregano, black pepper, red pepper flakes, salt, dried thyme)

Splenda
Vanilla
Wheat bran
Wheat germ
Whole wheat flour

BREAKFAST FOODS
All-Bran Buds cereal
Oatmeal (large-flake oats)

BEVERAGES
White wine

DAIRY CASE
Babybel Gouda Lite cheese
Buttermilk
Cheddar cheese (low-fat)
Cottage cheese (1%)
Fruit yogurt (non-fat with sweetener)
Laughing Cow Light cheese
Liquid eggs (e.g., Naturegg Break Free)
Milk (skim)
Mozzarella cheese (part-skim)
Plain yogurt (non-fat)
Soft margarine (non-hydrogenated, light)
Sour cream (low-fat)
Whole omega-3 eggs

FROZEN FOODS
Mixed berries
Peas (or fresh)

Week 10

Your Health—
What's at Stake

This week's topic follows from last week's discussion of motivation, since one of the top motivating factors for losing weight, as we saw in Week 1, is wanting to achieve better health. The connection between being overweight and being at increased risk for certain diseases is well established. Let's look at these risks in turn.

Heart Disease and Stroke

Given that I was the president of the Heart and Stroke Foundation of Ontario for fifteen years, it is hardly surprising that I'm starting with these diseases. However, there is a more important reason: heart disease and stroke cause 40 percent of North American deaths. Remarkably this is evidence of progress. When I first joined the foundation, the figure was close to 50 percent.

This is a good news/bad news story. The good news is that advances in surgery, drug therapies and emergency services have saved many lives. The bad news is that twice as many deaths could have been averted if only we had reduced our weight, exercised regularly and quit smoking. Though the smoking rate for adults has dropped sharply (unfortunately, we cannot say the same for teens), we are eating more and exercising less, leading inevitably to a more obese and unhealthy population. It has been calculated that if we led even a moderate lifestyle, we could halve the carnage from these diseases. Though heart disease, like most cancers, is primarily a disease of old age, nearly half of those who suffer heart attacks are under the age of sixty-five.

A familiar refrain that I have heard many times is "Why worry? If I have a heart attack, today's medicine will save me." It might well save you from immediate death, but the heart is permanently damaged after an attack. The heart cannot repair itself, because its cells do not reproduce. After the damage sustained during a heart attack, the heart has to work harder to compensate—but it never can. It slowly degenerates under this stress, and patients finally "drown" as blood circulation fails and the lungs fill with liquid. Congestive heart failure is a dreadful way to die, so make sure you do everything you can to avoid having a heart attack in the first place.

The simple fact is that the more overweight you are, the more likely you will suffer a heart attack or stroke. The two key factors that link heart disease and stroke to diet are cholesterol and hypertension (high blood pressure). High blood pressure puts more stress on the arterial system, causing it to age and deteriorate more rapidly, and ultimately leads to arterial damage, blood clots and heart attack or stroke. Excess weight has a major bearing on high blood pressure. One Canadian study found that obese adults aged eighteen to fifty-five had a five to thirteen times greater risk of hypertension. A further study demonstrated that a lower-fat diet coupled with a major increase in fruits and vegetables (eight to ten servings a day) lowered blood pressure. The moral: lose weight and eat more fruits and vegetables to help reduce your blood pressure levels. In other words, eat the green-light way.

Cholesterol is essential to your body's metabolism. However, high cholesterol is a problem, as it's the key ingredient in the plaque that can build up in your arteries, eventually cutting off the blood supply to your heart (causing heart attack) or your brain (leading to stroke). To make things more complicated, there are two forms of cholesterol: HDL (good) cholesterol and LDL (bad) cholesterol. (Remember it this way: HDL is Heart's Delight Level and LDL is Leads to Death Level.) The idea is to boost the HDL level while depressing the LDL level.

The villain in raising LDL levels is saturated fat, which is usually solid at room temperature and is found primarily in meat and whole milk products. Conversely, polyunsaturated and monounsaturated fats not only lower LDL levels but also boost HDL. The moral: make sure some fat is included in your diet, but make sure it's the right fat (see pages 10–12).

Diabetes

Diabetes is the kissing cousin of heart disease in that more people die from heart complications arising from diabetes than from diabetes alone. And diabetes rates are skyrocketing: they are expected to double in the next ten years.

The principal causes of the most common form of diabetes, type 2, are obesity and lack of exercise, and the current epidemic is strongly correlated to the obesity trend. The most dramatic illustration of this link appears in Canada's Native population, where in some communities diabetes affects nearly half the adults. Before the Europeans colonized North America, the Native peoples lived in a state of feast or famine. When there was an abundance of food, plant or animal, it was stored in the body as fat. In lean times, such as winter, the body depleted these fat supplies. As a result, their bodies developed a "thrift gene," with those who stored and utilized their food most effectively being the survivors—a classic Darwinian example of survival of the fittest. When you take away famine and the need to hunt or to harvest food—that is, the need to exercise—and replace it with a trip to the supermarket whenever food is required, the result is inevitable: a massive increase in obesity and, with it, diabetes.

Foods with a low G.I. rating, which release sugar more slowly into the bloodstream, appear to play a major role in helping diabetics control their disease. Thus, the G.I. Diet provides an opportunity both to lose weight and to assist in the management of the disease. In its magazine, *Dialogue,* the Canadian Diabetes Association selected the G.I. Diet as its diet of choice. Because protein and fat affect a food's G.I. rating, people with diabetes should be particularly careful about eating the right balance of green-light protein, carbohydrates and fat at every meal and snack. Prevention, however, is far preferable, so keep going with your green-light program and continue to slim down.

Cancer

There is increasing research evidence that diets high in saturated fat are linked to certain cancers, particularly prostate and colorectal cancer. A recent global report by the American Institute for Cancer Research concluded that 30 to 40 percent of cancers are directly linked to dietary choices. Its key recommendation is that individuals should choose a diet that includes a variety of vegetables, fruit and grains, and is low in saturated fat—in a nutshell, the G.I. Diet.

Alzheimer's Disease

As with cancer, there is increasing evidence linking certain dementias, particularly Alzheimer's, with fat intake. A recent U.S. study showed a 40 percent increase in Alzheimer's disease for those who ate a diet high in saturated fat.

Abdominal Fat and Health

Although your BMI is a measure of body fat based on your height and weight, it is not necessarily the best guide for assessing your health risk. Where you're storing the fat is the real issue. The results of a recent worldwide survey involving 27,000 people showed that people who carried their extra weight around their waists (apple shaped) were at far greater risk of disease than those who carried their weight lower down on their hips (pear shaped). From the study came this table showing the risk of disease based on weight and waist measurement.

WEIGHT	BMI	WAIST	WAIST
		Women less than 35'' Men less than 40''	Women 35'' plus MEN 40''plus
Normal	18.0–24.9	No risk increase	No risk increase
Overweight	25.0–29.9	Increased risk	High risk
Obese	30.0–39.9	High risk	Very high risk

A "beer belly" is not just extra weight. Rather, it is an active, living part of your body. Once it has formed sufficient mass, it behaves like an organ such as the liver, heart or kidney, except that it pumps out a dangerous combination of free fatty acids and proteins. The fact is that abdominal fat has many of the characteristics of a huge tumour. A waist measurement of 35 inches or more for women and 40 inches or more for men puts you in the High Risk category for developing heart disease, stroke, hypertension (high blood pressure) and certain types of cancer—breast, uterus, colon for women, and prostate and colon for men.

A further refinement, and an even better predictor of your health, is your waist-to-hip ratio. This is calculated by dividing your waist measurement by your hip measurement. A healthy ratio for women is 0.85 or below, and 0.95 or below for men. If you are a woman with a hip measurement of 42 inches and a waist measurement of 38 inches, your waist to hip ratio is 0.90, which puts you at risk. If your hip measurement was still 42 inches but your waist was only 34 inches, however, your ratio would be an acceptable 0.80.

Joint Degeneration

Finally, there is the issue of joint degeneration caused by excessive weight loading. Just recently, the Canadian Institute of Health published a survey of knee and hip replacements performed in Canada between 2004 and 2005. It showed that not only had the number of operations nearly doubled over the past ten years, but also that overweight patients accounted for a startling 87 percent of knee replacements and 74 percent of hip replacements.

If you want to reduce your risk for these diseases and keep your joints intact, then keep up your green-light diet. I can't think of a better motivator.

Week 10 Weight: _____

Week 10 Waist: _____

Week 10 Hips: _____

Week 10 Diary

Week 10 Optional Meal Plan

	BREAKFAST	SNACK	LUNCH	SNACK	DINNER	SNACK
MON	Homey Oatmeal (p. 204) with chopped apple	Carrot Muffin (p. 272)	Open-face lean deli ham sandwich with lettuce, tomato, red pepper and grainy mustard, and Basic G.I. Salad (p. 221)	Laughing Cow cheese with crispbread	Fettuccine Primavera (p. 231) and Caesar Salad (p. 222)	Mixed berries tossed in lime juice with sour cream
TUES	Mini Breakfast Puffs (p. 208)	Fruit yogurt	Waldorf Chicken and Rice Salad (p. 228)	Hummus with carrot and celery sticks	Ginger Wasabi Halibut (p. 246), Cold Noodle Salad with Cucumber and Sesame (p. 224), snow peas and carrots	Orange and almonds
WED	Homemade Muesli (p. 205) with skim milk and fruit yogurt	Carrot Muffin (p. 272)	Cottage cheese with apple and grapes, and Basic G.I. Salad (p. 221)	Babybel Gouda Lite cheese with crispbread	Chicken Tarragon with Mushrooms (p. 256) broccoli and basmati rice	Pecan Brownie (p. 283) and glass of skim milk
THURS	Homey Oatmeal (p. 204) with blueberries	Small apple and glass of skim milk	Minestrone Soup, (p. 214) and Basic G.I. Salad (p. 221)	Crunchy Chickpeas (p. 270)	Meatloaf (p. 261), green beans, carrots and new potatoes	1/2 nutrition bar
FRI	All-Bran Buds with skim milk, peach slices, and sliced almonds	Fruit yogurt	1/2 whole wheat pita with deli turkey, lettuce, tomato and cucumber, and Basic G.I. Salad (p. 221)	Laughing Cow cheese with crispbread	Bean and Onion Pizza (p. 235)	Mixed berries tossed in lime juice with sour cream
SAT	Italian Omelette (p. 210)	1/2 nutrition bar	Crab Salad in Tomato Shells (p. 229)	Hummus with carrot and celery sticks	Grilled Tuna with Chimichurri Sauce (p. 247), asparagus, and new potatoes	Pecan Brownie (p. 283) and glass of skim milk
SUN	Cinnamon French Toast (p. 206), with back bacon	Orange and almonds	Ham and Lentil Soup (p. 217), and Basic G.I. Salad (p. 221)	Babybel Gouda Lite cheese crispbread	Orange Chicken with Almonds (p. 255) green beans and basmati rice	Slice of Apple Raspberry Coffee Cake (p. 279)

Week 10 Grocery List for Meal Plan

PRODUCE
Almonds (whole and sliced)
Apples
Asparagus
Baby spinach
Bell peppers (red and green)
Blueberries (fresh or frozen)
Broccoli
Carrots
Celery
Cucumbers (English and field)
Fresh herbs (basil, chives, cilantro, flat-leaf
  parsley)
Garlic
Ginger root
Grapes
Green beans
Green onions
Lemon
Lettuce (leaf and Romaine)
Limes
Mushrooms
Onions (yellow and red)
Oranges
Peaches (fresh or canned in juice or water)
Pecans
Potatoes (new, small)
Raisins
Raspberries
Sesame seeds
Snow peas
Strawberries
Sun-dried tomatoes
Sunflower seeds, shelled and unsalted
Tofu (firm)
Tomatoes (large beefsteak and plum)
Walnuts
Zucchini (yellow)

DELI
Feta cheese (light)
Hummus (light)
Lean deli ham
Lean deli turkey
Parmesan cheese, grated

BAKERY
100% stone-ground whole wheat bread
Crispbread (e.g., Wasa Fibre)
Whole wheat pita bread

FISH COUNTER
Frozen crab
Halibut fillets
Tuna steaks ($1/2$-inch thick)

MEAT COUNTER
Back bacon
Chicken breasts (boneless, skinless)
Ground beef (extra-lean)

**BEANS (LEGUMES) AND
CANNED VEGETABLES**
Chickpeas
Kidney beans (red and white)
Lentils
Plum tomatoes
Tomato purée

PASTA AND SAUCES
Capellini or spaghettini (whole wheat)
Fettuccini or linguine (whole wheat)
Small pasta (e.g., ditali or tubetti)
Low-fat pasta sauce

SOUP AND CANNED SEAFOOD AND MEAT

Anchovy fillets
Chicken stock (low-fat, low-sodium)
Vegetable stock (low-fat, low-sodium)

GRAINS AND SIDE DISHES

Basmati rice
Flaxseeds

INTERNATIONAL FOODS

Mirin (or sweet sherry)
Rice vinegar
Soy sauce (low-sodium)
Sesame seeds (toasted)
Tahini
Wasabi powder

COOKING OIL, VINEGAR, SALAD DRESSINGS AND PICKLES

Buttermilk salad dressing (low-fat, low-sugar)
Dijon mustard
Grainy mustard
Oil (canola and extra-virgin olive)
Vegetable cooking oil spray (canola or olive oil)
Red wine vinegar
Worcestershire sauce

SNACKS

Nutrition bars (e.g., ZonePerfect, Balance Bar)

BAKING

Active dry yeast
Baking powder
Baking soda
Brown sugar substitute
Cornstarch
Oat bran
Spices (cayenne pepper, ground cinnamon, ground ginger, ground nutmeg, dried oregano, black pepper, red pepper flakes, salt, dried tarragon, dried thyme)
Splenda
Unsweetened cocoa powder
Vanilla
Wheat bran
Wheat germ
Whole wheat flour

BREAKFAST FOODS

All-Bran Buds cereal
Oatmeal (large-flake oats)

BEVERAGES

Tomato juice
Vegetable cocktail juice
Vermouth or white wine

DAIRY CASE

Babybel Gouda Lite cheese
Buttermilk
Fruit yogurt (non-fat with sweetener)
Laughing Cow Light cheese
Liquid eggs (e.g., Naturegg, Break Free)
Milk (skim)
Mozzarella cheese (part-skim)
Soft margarine (non-hydrogenated, light)
Sour cream (low-fat)
Whole omega-3 eggs

FROZEN FOODS SECTION

Peas (or fresh)
Mixed berries

Week 11

Holidays and
Special Events

Holidays are undoubtedly the most difficult times of the year for anyone trying to lose weight. While it may not actually be the holiday season when you come to this chapter, its advice can be applied to any sort of celebratory occasion, such as an anniversary, wedding or bar mitzvah. And of course you can always turn to this chapter when you are faced with the challenge of an approaching holiday. Celebrations like Thanksgiving, Easter, Passover and Christmas all have an abundance of food, and much of it is red-light. Many people gain weight as they indulge in the feasts at family get-togethers, office cocktail parties and neighbours' open houses, but it doesn't have to be this way. You can enjoy all the festivities and still stay mostly in the green. While it is probably unrealistic to expect you will lose weight during holiday time, your goal should be to not put on any more weight—after all, you've worked hard to achieve the progress you've made and you don't want to undo it! Here are my suggestions for navigating this dangerous terrain.

The Cocktail Party

Never go to a cocktail party hungry or you are likely to overindulge. Instead, have a small green-light meal or snack before heading out. A bowl of high-fibre green-light cereal will do the trick.

Once you arrive, be sure to get yourself a drink. It's important to always have a drink in hand at a cocktail party; if you don't, someone will probably pass you one that you haven't chosen—or you'll be looking for nibbles to occupy your empty hands. Soda water with a twist of lime or diet caffeine-free soft drinks are green-light choices. If you really would like an alcoholic beverage, bypass the beer and fancy cocktails, which are caloric nightmares, and instead choose a white wine spritzer or a glass of red wine. Try to limit yourself to one, and then switch to soda water.

Be sure to consume any alcohol with food to slow the rate at which you metabolize it. Look for green-light snacks such as mixed raw vegetables with low-fat dips such as hummus and salsa, lean sliced turkey and deli ham, shrimp (not breaded), smoked salmon, and fruit. Do not station yourself beside the bowls of nuts and olives—they may be green-light, but restricting yourself to a small handful will prove difficult.

The Holiday Dinner

It's easy to make your traditional festive meal green-light with some minor adjustments. Here are some guidelines:

Soup: Start the meal with a delicious, homemade green-light soup made with stock, vegetables and fresh herbs.

Salad: Always serve a large salad with homemade green-light dressing. Make it more festive by adding toasted pecans and a sprinkling of dried cranberries or crumbled blue cheese. Ruth makes a delicious salad of romaine lettuce, sliced strawberries and raspberry vinaigrette. Super easy and very pretty. The salad can be served before the main course to help fill you up, or as one of the side dishes.

Turkey: Prepare a roast turkey and eat the white breast meat—without the skin, of course. Instead of making stuffing with bread crumbs, use wild or basmati rice flavoured with apples or mushrooms, celery, onions and herbs.

Vegetables: There is a wide array of green-light vegetable dishes to choose from. Try roasted, braised or steamed vegetables in various combinations with flavourings of lemon, balsamic vinegar or herbs.

Sweet potatoes: If you consider sweet potatoes an essential part of your holiday feast, then go ahead and have them, but instead of adding brown sugar or maple syrup, try ground ginger, light non-hydrogenated margarine, pepper and hot water, if needed.

Cranberry sauce: If you make cranberry sauce, replace sugar with Splenda. Ruth always adds some chopped orange and slivered almonds for extra flavour and crunch.

Dessert: Dessert can always be part of a green-light meal. All of my books contain recipes for delicious desserts. A sweet treat to end your holiday dinner could be a low-fat, no-sugar-added ice cream, fresh berries with sweetened yogurt cheese, poached pears or a fruit crumble.

Hosting the holiday dinner yourself will obviously give you far greater control over the food. However, as a visitor, you can still exert some influence by bringing a green-light side dish or dessert and serving yourself. Compose your plate as you would at home: vegetables on half the plate, rice or pasta on one-quarter and a source of protein on the other quarter. Pass on the rolls and mashed potatoes—have extra vegetables instead. If you wish, you can allow yourself a concession by having a small serving of dessert. If you don't have much of a sweet tooth, you might prefer to have a glass of wine instead. Try not to indulge in both.

Here are some ways e-Clinic participants dealt with the holidays:

> "The newest strategy for our Christmas preparation is to focus on establishing new traditions with decorating and doing specific things together instead of the classics from my past that revolved around Christmas treats, such as Toblerone, chocolate oranges, Christmas cake and so on." —Bernadette

> "Thanksgiving went fairly well, with boiled new potatoes instead of mashed and smaller portions of white meat only and no seconds." —Ross

> "I was pleasantly surprised to get on the scales this morning and find I still weighed the same! One of the things I noticed yesterday was I was not left with that sick, stuffed feeling after the Thanksgiving meal! My biggest challenges were not tasting as I cooked the meal and deciding what to do with the leftovers, which I didn't want to waste. Would I rather they go to my waist? NOT! I gave away over half of them. We will have a few sensible meals out of the healthier ones. Some I simply dumped! Yay!" —Diane

> "Events such as Thanksgiving, Halloween and birthdays were always a 'free' ticket to overeat for me—it was almost as though it was expected. This time was different. I still enjoyed the food and celebrations, but when tempted to slide I thought, 'Is it worth having to wait another week or two or more to get to my goal?' I think more now

about what I am going to eat and why, especially if I'm out. I realize now what a lot of junk we feed ourselves. I wish that parents of young children would recognize this and take action, because they don't truly understand (and can't unless they have been there and lived it themselves) the impact that being overweight will have on their child emotionally, psychologically and physically, and the social stigma they will face." —Kathy

"This weekend was THE weekend for us for holiday parties. Friday night, Saturday lunch, Saturday night and Sunday lunch, followed by concert and dessert reception . . . I made myself a deal to cope with the events (I had no control over the food available): If I could eat mostly green- and some yellow-light foods, I could have a drink or two. If there were only yellow- or red-light foods available, it was club soda and lime for me." —Karen

Week 11 Weight: _____

Week 11 Waist: _____

Week 11 Hips: _____

Week 11 Diary

_____

_____

_____

_____

_____

_____

_____

_____

_____

_____

_____

_____

_____

_____

_____

_____

_____

_____

_____

_____

Week 11 Optional Meal Plan

	BREAKFAST	SNACK	LUNCH	SNACK	DINNER	SNACK
MON	Homey Oatmeal (p. 204) with chopped apple	Apple Bran Muffin (p. 273)	Open-face chicken sandwich with lettuce, tomato and onion, and Basic G.I. Salad (p. 221)	Laughing Cow Light cheese with crispbread	Rigatoni with Mini Meatballs (p. 284) and Caesar Salad (p. 222)	Mixed berries tossed in lime juice with sour cream
TUES	Mini Breakfast Puffs (p. 208)	Fruit yogurt	G.I. Pasta Salad (p. 225)	Hummus with carrot and celery sticks	Citrus-Poached Haddock (p. 245), green beans and new potatoes	Orange and almonds
WED	Homemade Muesli (p. 205) with skim milk and fruit yogurt	Apple Bran Muffin (p. 273)	1/2 whole wheat pita with canned light tuna, lettuce, tomato and cucumber, and Basic G.I. Salad (p. 221)	Babybel Gouda Lite cheese with crispbread	Chicken Jambalaya (p. 254) and broccoli	Creamy Lemon Square (p. 284) and glass of skim milk
THURS	Homey Oatmeal (p. 204) with blueberries	Small apple and glass of skim milk	Quick and Easy Chicken Noodle Soup (p. 216) and Basic G.I. Salad (p. 221)	Crunchy Chickpeas (p. 270)	Barley Risotto with Leeks, Lemon and Peas (p. 232), and Tabbouleh Salad (p. 226)	1/2 Nutrition bar
FRI	All-Bran Buds with skim milk, peach slices and sliced almonds	Fruit yogurt	Mixed Bean Salad (p. 227)	Laughing Cow Light cheese with crispbread	Thai Red Curry Shrimp Pasta (p. 243)	Mixed berries tossed in lime juice with sour cream
SAT	Vegetarian Omelette (p. 211)	1/2 nutrition bar	Greek Salad (p. 223)	Hummus with carrot and celery sticks	Zesty Barbecued Chicken (p. 258) Tangy Red and Green Coleslaw (p. 220) and new potatoes	Creamy Lemon Square (p. 284) and glass of skim milk
SUN	Oatmeal Buttermilk Pancakes (p. 207) with strawberries	Orange and almonds	Tuscan White Bean Soup (p. 215), and Basic G.I. Salad (p. 221)	Babybel Gouda Lite cheese with crispbread	Pork Tenderloin with Apple Compote (p. 268), Brussels sprouts, carrots and new potatoes	Piece of Berry Crumble (p. 277)

Week 11 Grocery List for Meal Plan

PRODUCE
Almonds (whole and sliced)
Apples
Bell peppers (red and green)
Blueberries (fresh or frozen)
Broccoli
Brussels sprouts
Cabbage (green and red)
Carrots
Celery
Cucumbers
Currants
Eggplant
Fresh herbs (chives, cilantro, flat-leaf parsley,
    mint, rosemary, sage and thyme)
Garlic
Green beans
Green onions
Kale
Leek
Lemons
Lettuce (leaf, iceberg and Romaine)
Limes
Mushrooms
Onions (yellow and red)
Oranges
Peaches (fresh or canned in juice or water)
Pecans
Potatoes (new, small)
Strawberries
Sunflower seeds, shelled and unsalted
Tomatoes (plum)
Zucchini

DELI
Feta cheese (light)
Hummus (light)

Kalamata olives
Parmesan cheese, grated

BAKERY
100% stone-ground whole wheat bread
Crispbread (e.g., Wasa Fibre)
Whole wheat pita bread

FISH COUNTER
Haddock fillets
Shrimp (large raw)

MEAT COUNTER
Chicken breasts (boneless, skinless)
Lean ground chicken or turkey
Pork tenderloin

BEANS (LEGUMES) AND
CANNED VEGETABLES
Chickpeas
Kidney beans (red and white)
Mixed beans
Plum tomatoes
Stewed tomatoes
Tomato paste

PASTA AND SAUCES
Rotini or penne (whole wheat)
Marcaroni or small shells (whole wheat)
Rigatoni (whole wheat)
Spagettini or linguine (whole wheat)
Small pasta (e.g., ditali or tubetti)
Light tomato sauce

SOUP AND CANNED SEAFOOD AND MEAT
Anchovy fillets
Chicken stock (low-fat, low-sodium)

Tuna (light, in water)
Vegetable stock (low-fat, low-sodium)

GRAINS AND SIDE DISHES
Barley
Brown rice
Bulgur
Flaxseeds

INTERNATIONAL FOODS
Tahini
Thai red curry paste

COOKING OIL, VINEGAR, SALAD DRESSINGS AND PICKLES
Cider vinegar
Dijon mustard
Mayonnaise (fat-free)
Oil (canola and extra-virgin olive)
Red wine vinegar
Vegetable cooking oil spray (canola or olive oil)
Worcestershire sauce

SNACKS
Applesauce (unsweetened)
Nutrition bars (e.g., ZonePerfect, Balance Bar)

BAKING
Baking powder
Baking soda
Brown sugar substitute
Cornstarch
Ground almonds
Oat bran
Spices (ground allspice, bay leaves, cayenne pepper, celery seeds, chili powder, ground cinnamon, ground cloves, ground cumin, dried oregano, black pepper, dried sage, salt, dried thyme)

Splenda
Vanilla
Wheat bran
Wheat germ
Whole wheat flour

BREAKFAST FOODS
All-Bran Buds cereal
Oatmeal (large-flake oats)

BEVERAGES
Apple juice (unsweetened)
Dry white wine (or vermouth)

DAIRY CASE
Babybel Gouda Lite cheese
Buttermilk
Cheddar cheese (low-fat)
Fruit yogurt (non-fat with sweetener)
Laughing Cow Light cheese
Liquid eggs (e.g., Naturegg, Break Free)
Milk (skim)
Orange juice (unsweetened)
Soft margarine (non-hydrogenated, light)
Sour cream (low-fat)
Whole omega-3 eggs

FROZEN FOODS
Frozen apple juice concentrate
Mixed berries
Peas (or fresh)

Week 12

Exercise

As the e-Clinic progressed and participants lost a considerable amount of weight and found their energy level increasing, many decided to get involved in regular exercise.

> "Now that eating is becoming more routine, I want to establish an exercise program. I think this will be important." —Lynn

> "I can almost see the 100s and I am dying to get there! . . . I joined Curves (a fitness club) yesterday." —Beverley

> "I am down below what I have been for the past seven years. That is encouraging and I know I will continue the good eating habits I have practised for the last three months. I also know I am at a place where I need to increase my daily exercise." —Diane

> "When my baby was six months old, I tried jogging but was discouraged when I felt a lot of pain in my shins. This past Thursday, I tried it again and had great success. I have jogged almost every day so far." —Tammy

There are many benefits to exercising. Regular exercise will contribute significantly to your health by reducing your risk of heart disease, stroke, diabetes and osteoporosis; maintaining your muscle mass and tone as you age; and, over the long term, accelerating or maintaining your weight loss. In the United States, the National Weight Loss Registry is tracking some 3000 people who have lost 30 pounds or more and kept it off for six years. One thing they have in common is that they are very active and exercise every day. Although exercise is of limited value in helping you achieve your weight-loss target, it becomes a critical factor in helping you maintain your weight and health for the rest of your life. And believe it or not, exercise can become addictive. I tend to become irritable and edgy if I'm not getting my daily exercise fix—or so Ruth tells me. Initially it can be hard to get out there and hit the sidewalk or gym, but stick with it—the fun will kick in eventually.

Types of Exercise

Before we go any further, we should define exactly what we mean by exercise. There are three basic types of exercise, each working with the others.

Aerobic

Aerobic exercise gets your heart and lungs working harder. Aerobic exercise, such as walking, jogging, biking, swimming, hiking and so on, will have the most impact on your overall weight and health.

Strength

Strength training is particularly important as we move into middle age and beyond because of the steady reduction in muscle mass that accompanies aging. Starting at the age of twenty-five, the body loses 2 percent of its muscle mass each decade, a process that accelerates to 6 to 8 percent as we move into our senior years.

Exercising muscles on a regular basis minimizes or reverses the loss. And why is that important? Because the larger your muscles, the more energy (calories) they use. When you're at rest, or even asleep in bed, your muscles are using energy. So keeping or building muscle mass really helps you burn calories and lose weight.

Though regular exercise will help minimize muscle loss, it is through resistance exercises that we actually build muscle mass. Resistance exercises involve fixed or free weights, elastic bands or even your own body weight; pushing your hands together as hard as you can is a form of resistance exercise. You don't have to join a gym or work out with massive barbells. A few simple exercises, easily done at home, will do wonders to restore or tone those flabby muscles.

Stretching

Again, this is a significant issue as we age and lose flexibility in our joints, tendons and ligaments. Loss of flexibility reduces our ability to do either aerobic or strength training, both of which depend on healthy joints and tissues. In older people, this loss of flexibility can lead to falls and hip fractures. So although stretching may seem like a "frill," it is central to the whole fitness picture.

Stretching exercises will also give you the biggest bang for your buck in terms of immediate payout. Within just a week, you can increase your flexibility by over 100 percent. Both aerobic exercise and strength training can actually make you less flexible if you don't stretch those muscle ligaments and tendons. That's why you always see athletes warming up and down with stretching exercises. Always include stretching in your exercise program.

Now let's review your options.

Outdoor Activities

Walking

This is by far the simplest and, for most people, the easiest exercise program to start and maintain. For adults, thirty minutes a day, seven days a week, should be the target. If you do an hour-long walk one day of the weekend, you can take a day off during the week. We're talking about brisk walking, neither speed walking nor ambling along. Imagine you're late for an appointment, and keep that pace. You should increase your heart and breathing rates, but never to the point where you lack the breath to talk with a partner.

You don't need any special clothing or equipment, except a pair of comfortable cushioned shoes or running shoes. Walking is rarely boring since you can change routes and watch the world go by. Walk with your spouse, child or friend for company and mutual support, or go solo and commune with nature and your own thoughts. I prefer to walk on my own in the morning, which is when I do my best thinking. This is not surprising when you realize how much extra oxygen-fresh blood is pumping through the brain.

A great idea for working people is to incorporate walking into the daily commute. I used to get off the bus three stops early on my way to and from work. Those three stops are equal to about $1^1/2$ miles, so I was walking about 3 miles per day! If you drive to work, try parking your car a few blocks away and walk to your job. You may even find cheaper parking. Gradually increase the distance and your exercise. Who knows, you may eventually be able to walk to work. Think of the savings in gas and parking fees!

Jogging

This is similar to walking, but you need the proper footwear to protect joints from damage. Jogging approximately doubles the number of calories burned in the same period of time as walking: 400 calories for jogging versus 200 for brisk walking over a thirty-minute period. While walking, try jogging for a few yards and see if it is for you. Jogging increases your heart rate, which is great for heart health. Like all muscles, the heart thrives on exercise so, in general, the more the better. If jogging suits you, then this could be the simplest and most effective method of exercise as it can be done anywhere and is inexpensive.

Hiking

Another variation on walking is cross-country hiking. Because this usually involves different kinds of terrain, especially hills and valleys, you use more calories, about 50 percent more than for brisk walking. Try hauling 150 to 200 pounds up a hill and you'll get some idea of the extra effort your body has to make.

Bicycling

Like walking, jogging and hiking, bicycling is a fun way to burn calories, and it is almost as effective as jogging (for people with low-back or knee problems, it can be preferable). Other than the cost of the bike and helmet, it's inexpensive and can be done almost anywhere, with lights and reflectors for night riding, of course.

Sports

Although most sports are terrific calorie burners, they usually cannot be part of a regular routine. Most of them require other people, equipment and facilities. But they can provide a boost to your regular fitness and exercise program. Such popular sports as tennis, basketball, soccer, softball and golf (no golf cart, please) are excellent additions to a basic exercise program. However, they're no substitute for a five- to seven-day-a-week regular schedule.

Indoor Activities

Many of you will be muttering by now about how this would be fine advice if we lived in California. But many of us must contend with either frigid, snowy winters or hot, humid summers, which limit outdoor activities.

The alternatives are either to organize a home gym or join a fitness club. The advantage of clubs is that they offer a wide range of sophisticated equipment, with instruction and advice from staff. Clubs are also social, and some people find they need group motivation to work out with enthusiasm. YMCA/YWCAs and some community centres also offer special programs for elderly people, new mothers, and those with special needs; some provide subsidies for people who can't afford the membership fees. Many centres offer free fitness classes too.

If a fitness club isn't convenient or those Lycra-clad young things make you uncomfortable, you can always set up an exercise area at home. The best and least expensive piece of equipment is a stationary bike. The latest models work on magnetic resistance rather than the old friction strap around the flywheel. This gives a smoother action, with better tension adjustment. Most important, they are quiet, which is crucial if you want to be able to listen to music or watch TV.

You can easily pay in the thousands for a bike with all the fancy trimmings, but the $250 to $300 machines will work fine. Just be sure you choose one that has smooth, adjustable tension; then pop in that late-night movie or your favourite soap and get pedalling. You'll be amazed how quickly the minutes fly by. Twenty minutes on the bike consumes the same number of calories as thirty minutes of brisk walking.

If biking is not for you, try a treadmill. These can be expensive, and beware of the lower-end models that cannot take the pounding. Expect to pay about $1,000 and up. Make sure the incline of the track can be raised and lowered for a better workout. Treadmills and bikes can simulate outdoor walking, jogging, hiking or biking in the comfort of your own home. I use both of these machines but have added a cross-country ski machine, which has the advantage of working the upper body as well. Ski machines are generally less expensive than treadmills, but cost more than stationary bikes. They also burn a lot of calories (similar to the amount burned when jogging) because they use the arms and shoulders as well as the legs. Ski machines are almost the perfect all-body workout machine.

There are several other specialized options, such as stair climber machines, elliptical walkers and rowing machines, but they're not for everyone. Many are also quite expensive, so try them out first at a fitness club or with a cooperative retailer.

Strength Training

It's now time to pay attention to rebuilding your muscle mass. Remember that, after age forty, you may lose between 4 and 6 pounds of muscle every decade, which is usually replaced with flab. That's 4 to 6 pounds of calorie-consuming muscle. Muscles burn energy even when idle, and bigger muscles consume more energy than smaller muscles. So muscles come in handy for losing or maintaining weight.

Resistance-training equipment can range from the complex and expensive to a $10 rubber band. Home gyms, with prices that begin at a couple of hundred dollars, are a popular option. For most people, however, there are cheaper, simpler methods, such as a set of free weights or (my own preference) rubber exercise bands. Dyna-Band and Thera-Band are two popular choices. I like using Thera-Bands, which come in varying thicknesses that offer increasing levels of resistance as you regain and build your muscle strength.

Weights and resistance rubber bands are available at many fitness exercise equipment retailers and surgical supply stores. Try a few resistance exercises, concentrating on the larger muscle groups—your legs, arms and upper chest. These are the muscles that will give you the biggest bang by burning up the most calories. Resistance exercises should complement your regular exercise regimen, not replace it. Committing to both types of exercise will produce far better results than either one alone. Resistance exercises are best done every other day, leaving time for your muscles to recuperate.

Pilates

I've recently become a Pilates enthusiast. Originally, it was recommended by my physiotherapist to strengthen my back and prevent my disc problem from recurring. However, this very precise system of exercises does a lot more than just that. It's a series of floor exercises—no equipment needed—that both strengthen and stretch your muscles, especially the core muscles in your back and around your waist, which are essential for good posture. It's great for any level of fitness and at any age.

Yoga and Tai Chi

Yoga comes in different styles: hatha, kundalini, kripalu, ashtanga, bikram and others. If you're new to yoga, the best choice is hatha, which teaches you simple postures that will keep you supple, relax you and improve your breathing and circulation. But in any form, this ancient practice has much to offer, especially to anyone taking up exercise in middle age.

Tai Chi is another Eastern discipline that is gentle, promoting flexibility, balance and energy. It features a series of flowing postures, done standing, that many people like to practise early in the morning, outdoors. Tai Chi keeps the joints and tendons supple, and offers a peaceful, revitalizing form of activity that can carry you into old age.

Instructional DVDs or videos are available for those who want to learn or practise yoga or Tai Chi at home.

For more suggestions about incorporating physical activity into your daily life, check out the Canadian Public Health Agency website at www.phac-aspc.gc.ca/pau-uap/fitness.

Whether you take up walking, hockey, dance lessons or nature hikes, make sure it is an activity you enjoy. If you take pleasure from your exercise, you are more likely to do it.

Week 12 Weight:_____

Week 12 Waist:_____

Week 12 Hips:_____

Week 12 Diary

_____

_____

_____

_____

_____

_____

_____

_____

_____

_____

_____

_____

_____

_____

_____

_____

_____

_____

Week 12 Optional Meal Plan

	BREAKFAST	SNACK	LUNCH	SNACK	DINNER	SNACK
MON	Homey Oatmeal (p. 204) with chopped apple	Whole Wheat Fruit Scone (p. 274)	Open-face lean deli ham sandwich with lettuce, tomato, red pepper and grainy mustard, and Basic G.I. Salad (p. 221)	Laughing Cow Light cheese with crispbread	Salmon Pasta (p. 242)	Mixed berries tossed in lime juice with sour cream
TUES	Mini Breakfast Puffs (p. 208)	Fruit yogurt	Waldorf Chicken and Rice Salad (p. 228)	Hummus with carrot and celery sticks	Pan-Seared White Fish with Mandarin Salsa (p. 248), broccoli and basmati rice	Orange and almonds
WED	Homemade Muesli (p. 205) with skim milk and fruit yogurt	Whole Wheat Fruit Scone (p. 274)	Cottage cheese with apple and grapes, and Basic G.I. Salad (p. 221)	Babybel Gouda Lite cheese with crispbread	Chicken Schnitzel (p. 253), green beans, carrots and new potatoes	Slice of Strawberry Tea Bread (p. 275) and glass of skim milk
THURS	Homey Oatmeal (p. 204) with blueberries	Small apple and glass of skim milk	Minestrone Soup (p. 214) and Basic G.I. Salad (p. 221)	Crunchy Chickpeas (p. 270)	Mushroom and Gravy Pork Chops (p. 267), asparagus and basmati rice	1/2 nutrition bar
FRI	All-Bran Buds with skim milk, peach slices and sliced almonds	Fruit yogurt	1/2 whole wheat pita with deli turkey, lettuce, tomato and cucumber, and Basic G.I. Salad (p. 221)	Laughing Cow Light cheese with crispbread	Horseradish Burgers (p. 262) and Tabbouleh Salad (p. 226)	Mixed berries tossed in lime juice with sour cream
SAT	Back Bacon Omelette (p. 209)	1/2 nutrition bar	Crab Salad in Tomato Shells (p. 229)	Hummus with carrot and celery sticks	Vegetarian Moussaka (p. 239) and basmati rice	Slice of Strawberry Tea Bread (p. 275) and glass of skim milk
SUN	Cinnamon French Toast (p. 206) with back bacon	Orange and almonds	Ham and Lentil Soup (p. 217) and Basic G.I. Salad (p. 221)	Babybel Gouda Lite cheese with crispbread	Spicy Roasted Chicken with Tomatoes and Tarragon (p. 256), green beans and basmati rice	Slice of One-Bowl Chocolate Cake (p. 281) with berries

Week 12 Grocery List for Meal Plan

PRODUCE
Alfalfa sprouts (optional)
Almonds (whole and sliced)
Apples
Asparagus
Baby spinach
Bell peppers (red and green)
Blueberries (fresh or frozen)
Broccoli
Carrots
Celery
Cucumbers
Dried apricots
Eggplants
Fresh herbs (basil, chives, cilantro, flat-leaf
   parsley, mint, tarragon)
Garlic
Grapes
Green beans
Green onions
Lemons
Lettuce (leaf)
Limes
Mushrooms
Onions (yellow and red)
Oranges
Peaches (fresh or canned in juice or water)
Pecans
Potatoes (new, small)
Strawberries
Sun-dried tomatoes
Sunflower seeds, shelled and unsalted
Tomatoes (large beefsteak, plum, and cherry
or grape)
Walnuts

DELI
Feta cheese (light)
Hummus (light)
Lean deli ham
Lean deli turkey
Light herb and garlic cream cheese
Parmesan cheese, grated

BAKERY
100% stone-ground whole wheat bread
Crispbread (e.g., Wasa Fibre)
Whole wheat breadcrumbs
Whole wheat hamburger buns
Whole wheat pita bread

FISH COUNTER
Frozen crab
Salmon fillet
White fish fillets

MEAT COUNTER
Back bacon
Boneless pork loin chops
Chicken breasts (boneless, skinless)
Ground beef (extra-lean)

**BEANS (LEGUMES) AND
CANNED VEGETABLES**
Chickpeas
Kidney beans (red)
Lentils
Diced tomatoes
Plum tomatoes
Tomato paste

PASTA AND SAUCES
Macaroni (whole wheat)
Small pasta (e.g., ditali or tubetti)

SOUP AND CANNED SEAFOOD AND MEAT
Chicken stock (low-fat, low-sodium)

GRAINS AND SIDE DISHES
Basmati rice
Bulgur

INTERNATIONAL FOODS
Rice vinegar

COOKING OIL, VINEGAR, SALAD DRESSINGS AND PICKLES
Buttermilk salad dressing (low-fat, low sugar)
Dijon mustard
Grainy mustard
Horseradish
Mayonnaise (fat-free)
Oil (canola and extra-virgin olive)
Red wine vinegar
Steak sauce
Vegetable cooking oil spray (canola or olive oil)
Worcestershire sauce

SNACKS
Applesauce (unsweetened)
Nutrition bars (e.g., ZonePerfect, Balance Bar)
Canned mandarin oranges (no added sugar)

BAKING
Baking powder
Baking soda
Oat bran
Spices (ground allspice, dried basil, cayenne pepper, ground cinnamon, ground cumin, Italian herb seasoning, nutmeg, dried oregano, black pepper, red pepper flakes, salt, dried thyme)
Splenda
Unsweetened cocoa powder

Vanilla
Wheat bran
Wheat germ
Whole wheat flour

BREAKFAST FOODS
All-Bran Buds cereal
Oatmeal (large-flake oats)

BEVERAGES
Apple juice (unsweetened)
Dry white wine (or vermouth)

DAIRY CASE
1% pressed cottage cheese
Babybel Gouda Lite cheese
Buttermilk
Fruit yogurt (non-fat with sweetener)
Laughing Cow Light cheese
Liquid eggs (e.g., Naturegg, Break Free)
Milk (skim)
Orange juice (unsweetened)
Soft margarine (non-hydrogenated, light)
Sour cream (low-fat)

FROZEN FOODS
Mixed berries
Peas (or fresh)

Week 13

When Weight
Loss Causes Anxiety

On this, the last week of your three-month journey on the G.I. Diet, I would like to talk about the influence of social factors on the weight-loss experience. Many e-Clinic participants told me that they didn't want their family, friends and co-workers to know they were trying to lose weight.

> "I have not told any co-workers and only two close friends about being on the program because of the fear of the 'I told you so,' 'I knew you'd never stick to it,' and 'You're on another diet?' responses I have heard all my life from my mother and others . . . Social situations are still uncomfortable for me and I am very self conscious about how I look."
> —Kathy

> "In group situations (especially with family), if I'm not eating what other people are eating, then people are going to talk. They're going to start asking me if I'm on a diet, and I don't want to admit that I am, because my low self-esteem says that I'm not going to be able to do it, and then everyone will talk about what a failure I am." —Lynette

> "I often feel self-conscious because of my size and appearance, so what better way to bury these bad feelings than with my old friend and comfort blanket: lots of food? Also, I avoid calling attention to myself by reverting to old eating patterns so no one asks why I'm not overeating as usual, in other words acting normal to avoid scrutiny."
> —Ross

Anxiety about being caught failing and feeling humiliated can be exacerbated when people start noticing your weight loss and ask questions like, "Have you lost some weight?" or "What diet are you trying now?" You might start to feel like you're being watched, and like people are wondering how long it will be before you give up. This is especially true if you have been a yo-yo dieter. The best defence in this case is to have a set of responses ready for their comments:

- "Thank you for noticing."
- "Thanks. I'm going to need your support as I do this. Let me tell you how you can help . . ."
- "I know you want me to succeed, so I can improve my health. Let me tell you how you can help . . ."

Family members can be the most discouraging. Here is an example from Pat:

> "When my sister met me to drive me home, she commented on how she could tell that I had lost a significant amount of weight. That made me feel great. I said, 'Oh that reminds me that I have some dress pants that are getting too big.' Her response was, 'Oh just put them in a box—you never know when you will need them again.' Horrified, I said I would never need them again. How is that for a little encouragement and discouragement all at the same time?"

If you become the target of dispiriting comments like, "So what's the magic diet this time round?" or "How long will the weight be off this time?" try squelching them with kindness. Say something like, "Jim, I'm sure you want me to succeed, so saying something supportive would be much more helpful." Then smile—you'll feel better for taking the high road.

There can be some hidden anxiety about changing your body. Strange though it may seem when your greatest wish is to be slim and trim, deep down you may worry that you won't recognize the new you and that you won't be the same person.

Does personality change when you lose weight? Certainly you may feel healthier, have more energy, sleep better, worry less and feel less depressed, but none of this has anything to do with your personality, which is formed early on and makes you unique and different from everyone else. Your personality is essentially who you are, and it's not going to change when you lose weight. If you have a wicked sense of humour, it's not going to disappear when you lose a hundred pounds. If you are shy, losing weight isn't going to turn you into a party animal. You may feel more comfortable in social situations, but you will still be you. Some of the defensive behaviours you developed to survive being large in the world may disappear with the pounds, but the fundamental you will remain.

Excess weight is often subconsciously used to hide and protect the body. Ironically, being large can make people "invisible"—that is, unnoticed or ignored. Excess weight can be a way to desexualize the body, in that men and women can lose their sexual attractiveness and gender-specific qualities. We know from research that women with eating disorders such as anorexia sometimes use starvation to lose all their female sexual characteristics. Large women may similarly be hiding theirs with fat. The reasons can be complex. Some women with histories of sexual abuse do this as a means of protection, believing that men will not be attracted to a large, asexual body. Losing excess weight can give the body a defined shape, making women look more feminine and men more masculine. They may suddenly be seen and noticed, and considered physically attractive or "sexy," which may be anxiety-producing. But the reality is that it is a whole lot easier living in this society when your body is not overweight. Slender people tend to be treated better than overweight people, and research shows that slender people are regarded as being brighter, richer and happier than those who are overweight. People who are attractive advance more quickly in the workplace.

Once you've lost a significant amount of weight and bought yourself a new wardrobe, start practising how you will behave in potentially anxiety-provoking situations. E-clinic participants wrote me about some awkward situations:

> "When people comment on my changing appearance . . . it is sometimes difficult to suppress that inner voice that tends to 'overthink' things, and this leads to misinterpretation of a simple compliment. There are undeniable emotionally laden aspects to this process that lead to veering off the path, so to speak." —Bernadette

> "So many people in my office have now bought your book (I bet at least nine people) and come to me regularly for help and guidance. It is so funny. They are all amazed at the physical transition. I wore low-waisted jeans last week and felt like a monkey in a zoo. People were coming by to look at me because someone else would say, 'Have you

seen Bev today? She looks great.' I found it a little embarrassing. I kept apologizing and saying, 'Well, I still have a lot to lose.' My girlfriend told me to accept it and just say thanks, because I've worked hard and it shows. (She is a big support)." —Beverley

Try to do some role-playing with a close friend. Have him or her comment on how good you look, pay you compliments, ask you out—whatever you might find difficult—and practise your responses. If someone comments on how good you look or likes your new outfit, practise looking them straight in the eye and saying thank you—no qualifying statements, please! In our politically correct world, it is unlikely anyone would dare tell you that you look "sexy," but if they do, figure out what light comment you could make before contemplating filing a complaint!

As you start to make friends with and become familiar with your new body, remember that virtually everyone is dissatisfied with their bodies—even those whose bodies seem perfect. They too are filled with self-doubt and look for that new lotion or potion that will improve how they look. Where would the beauty industry be without all our anxieties? So don't think you're the only one worrying while everyone else feels secure about themselves. We all wish we could be better somehow. Just enjoy your lighter body, and remember that the goal is not perfection, but a more comfortable and healthy self.

Well, dear reader, by now you have completed a three-month journey on the G.I. Diet. Some of you may have reached your target weight, while others will still have some way to go. In the next chapter, I will reveal the results achieved by some of our e-Clinic participants and include their thoughts on the program.

Week 13 Weight: _____

Week 13 Waist: _____

Week 13 Hips: _____

Week 13 Diary

_____

_____

_____

_____

_____

_____

_____

_____

_____

_____

_____

_____

_____

_____

_____

_____

_____

Week 13 Optional Meal Plan

	BREAKFAST	SNACK	LUNCH	SNACK	DINNER	SNACK
MON	Homey Oatmeal (p. 204) with chopped apple	Cranberry Cinnamon Bran Muffin (p. 271)	Open-face chicken sandwich with lettuce, tomato and onion and Basic G.I. Salad (p. 221)	Laughing Cow Light cheese with crispbread	Easy-Bake Lasagna (p. 237) and Caesar Salad (p. 222)	Mixed berries tossed in lime juice with sour cream
TUES	Mini Breakfast Puffs (p. 208)	Fruit yogurt	G.I. Pasta Salad (p. 225)	Hummus with carrot and celery sticks	G.I. Fish Fillet (p. 244), asparagus, carrots and new potatoes	Orange and almonds
WED	Homemade Muesli (p. 205) with skim milk and fruit yogurt	Cranberry Cinnamon Bran Muffin (p. 271)	1/2 whole wheat pita with canned light tuna, lettuce, tomato and cucumber, and Basic G.I. Salad (p. 221)	Babybel Gouda Lite cheese with crispbread	Chicken Curry (p. 252) and Raita Salad (p. 219)	Apple Pie Cookie (p. 282) and glass of skim milk
THURS	Homey Oatmeal (p. 204) with blueberries	Small apple and glass of skim milk	Quick and Easy Chicken Noodle Soup (p. 216) and Basic G.I. Salad (p. 221)	Crunchy Chickpeas (p. 270)	Vegetable Crumble (p. 233) and Tabbouleh Salad (p. 226)	1/2 nutrition bar
FRI	All-Bran Buds with skim milk, peach slices and sliced almonds	Fruit yogurt	Mixed Bean Salad (p. 227)	Laughing Cow Light cheese with crispbread	Chicken Fried Rice (p. 251)	Mixed berries tossed in lime juice with sour cream
SAT	Western Omelette (p. 212)	1/2 nutrition bar	Greek Salad (p. 223)	Hummus with carrot and celery sticks	Beef and Eggplant Chili (p. 263) and Basic G.I. Salad (p. 221)	Apple Pie Cookie (p. 282), and glass of skim milk
SUN	Oatmeal Buttermilk Pancakes (p. 207) with strawberries	Orange and almonds	Tuscan White Bean Soup (p. 215), and G.I. Salad (p. 221)	Babybel Gouda Lite cheese with Basic crispbread	Pork Medallions Dijon (p. 266), green beans, carrots and new potatoes	Piece of Plum Crumble (p. 278)

Week 13 Grocery List for Meal Plan

PRODUCE
Almonds (whole and sliced)
Apples
Asparagus
Baby spinach
Bean sprouts
Bell peppers (red and green)
Blueberries (fresh or frozen)
Broccoli
Carrots
Celery
Cranberries (dried)
Cucumbers (English and field)
Eggplant
Fresh herbs (chives, mint, flat-leaf parsley,
    sage, tarragon, thyme)
Garlic
Green beans
Green onions
Kale
Leeks
Lemons
Lettuce (iceberg, leaf and Romaine)
Mixed nuts
Mushrooms
Onions (yellow and red)
Oranges
Peaches (fresh or canned in juice or water)
Potatoes (new, small)
Prune plums (e.g., damson or Italian)
Raisins
Sesame seeds
Strawberries
Sunflower seeds shelled and unsalted
Sweet potato
Tofu (firm)
Tomatoes (plum)
Zucchini

DELI
Feta cheese (light)
Hummus (light)
Kalamata olives
Parmesan cheese, grated

BAKERY
100% stone-ground whole wheat bread
Crispbread (e.g., Wasa Fibre)
Whole wheat pita bread

FISH COUNTER
Fish fillets (salmon or trout)

MEAT COUNTER
Back bacon
Chicken breasts (boneless, skinless)
Ground beef (extra-lean)
Pork tenderloins

**BEANS (LEGUMES) AND
CANNED VEGETABLES**
Chickpeas
Kidney beans (red and white)
Mixed beans
Diced tomatoes
Plum tomatoes
Tomato paste

PASTA AND SAUCES
Lasagna (whole wheat)
Rotini or penne (whole wheat)
Small pasta (e.g., ditali or tubetti)
Light tomato sauce (no added sugar)
Low-fat pasta sauce

SOUP AND CANNED SEAFOOD AND MEAT
Anchovy fillets
Chicken stock (low-fat, low-sodium)
Tuna (light, in water)
Vegetable stock (low-fat, low-sodium)

GRAINS AND SIDE DISHES
Basmati rice
Brown rice
Bulgur
Flaxseeds

INTERNATIONAL FOODS
Sesame oil
Soy sauce (low-sodium)
Tahini

COOKING OIL, VINEGAR, SALAD DRESSINGS AND PICKLES
Dijon mustard
Mayonnaise (fat-free)
Oil (canola and extra-virgin olive)
Red wine vinegar
Vegetable cooking oil spray (canola or olive oil)
Worcestershire sauce

SNACKS
Applesauce (unsweetened)
Nutrition bars (e.g., ZonePerfect, Balance Bar)

BAKING
Baking powder
Baking soda
Cornstarch
Oat bran
Spices (ground cardamom, cayenne pepper, chili powder, ground cinnamon, ground cumin, curry powder, ground ginger, ground nutmeg, dried oregano, black pepper, red pepper flakes, salt, dried thyme)
Splenda
Vanilla
Wheat bran
Wheat germ
Whole wheat flour

BREAKFAST FOODS
All-Bran Buds cereal
Oatmeal (large-flake oats)

BEVERAGES
White wine

DAIRY CASE
Babybel Gouda Lite cheese
Buttermilk
Cheddar cheese (low-fat)
Cottage cheese (1%)
Fruit yogurt (non-fat with sweetener)
Laughing Cow Light cheese
Liquid eggs (e.g., Naturegg Break Free)
Milk (skim)
Mozzarella cheese (part-skim)
Plain yogurt (non-fat)
Soft margarine (non-hydrogenated, light)
Sour cream (low-fat)
Whole omega-3 eggs

FROZEN FOODS
Mixed berries
Peas (or fresh)

Results of the E-Clinic

I'm sure you're all wondering how everyone did after the first thirteen weeks of the e-Clinic. Well, I'm really delighted with the participants' overall progress. I'm happy to report that we had a dropout rate of less than 20 percent—and that includes those who had to leave the program for medical reasons, such as chemotherapy and hip replacement. Those who stayed with it lost significant amounts of weight. In this chapter, I will share with you the results of some of the participants as well as their comments about what they learned and experienced while on the program. Now of course the results varied from person to person, but this is in no way a reflection of their commitment or of their achievements—we all have different body shapes, metabolisms, ages and medical histories and we all lose weight at different rates. They all deserve a big pat on the back!

From Bernadette, who lost 20 pounds and a total of 8 inches from her waist and hips:

> "I can honestly say that I never felt hungry or deprived during the thirteen weeks. This is probably the most significant and critical difference from other weight-loss approaches that I have tried. Not having to measure and weigh most of the food that I eat has probably been the next most critical factor in the success that I have experienced to date.

Having to do that in the past with other weight-loss programs and then keep track of points was not compatible with real life and quickly gave way to resentment and failure.

"I do like that the range of choices is so broad in most categories of foods listed and that you don't have a feeling of restriction . . . I believe that the difference between success at this process of weight loss and failure is quickly overcoming a setback, whether it be making a bad choice or however you want to describe not sticking to the plan. I have come to understand that putting a setback behind you and getting quickly back on track is the key to success. Anything else just perpetuates that 'I blew it and what's the point' feeling and holds you back . . . I appreciate your support and I am excited about the continued feeling of vitality that I have rediscovered. For that I am very grateful."

From Diane, who lost 19 pounds:

"I am still a little disappointed with my total lost amount, but I know that I am down below what I have been for the past seven years. That is encouraging and I know I will continue the good eating habits I have practised for the last three months . . . I think that my husband and I have always practised pretty good 'home cooking' eating habits—we already used low-fat, sugar-free items and ate lean meats. But I have had a big problem with being a 'stress eater' and a 'social eater' (going out to restaurants, inviting people over, fast food convenience). You have helped me with these issues a lot! Having items for snacks has greatly helped! . . . I have so much more energy this season than I did a year ago. I can remember last year I didn't even want to put up my Christmas decorations because I just did not have the energy. This year, I feel back to my old self. Now I just need to find that self that I haven't seen since around 1995 (when I was diagnosed with asthma and started gaining my weight back)! I know I can do this—for me!

Thanks again! It has been a great three months!"

From Ross, who lost 46 pounds:

"One of the biggest obstacles I personally have found, besides all the usual ones, is poor planning as far as shopping goes. I would run out of green-light items and occasionally revert 'just this once' to red-light foods, as they were now quicker because 'I didn't have time to go shopping at the moment and needed to eat.' I now work out a plan for a week or so, listing the days and the meals and a possible menu . . . This takes only a few minutes to actually do the 'math' and write the list, plus of course, I have to actually get the shopping done."

From Karen, who lost 16 pounds and a total of 7 inches from her waist and hips:

"My biggest suggestion for others is to have as much green-light food around you as possible for the situations you CAN control. I can control my home and my office (meaning my immediate office, not the communal kitchen). I cannot control what is available when I am at other people's homes or the office cafeteria, which still serves meatloaf and mashed potatoes or pizza as your two hot choices! I can (however dorky it seems) bring two slices of high-fibre whole wheat bread in my purse, get the insides of my sandwich from the salad bar and make my own sandwich at the table. Restaurants take practice, but as you've said there are usually enough good choices to cobble together a meal. I've eaten out an average of three lunches and three dinners per week and still have lost weight. Of course, the weeks I brown bag it and eat dinner at home I have better results.

"I've also learned that I share my home and office with 'diet assassins.' I think they think if they can get me to cheat, it absolves their bad eating habits. Last night I found myself making chocolate chip cookies because my husband and co-workers requested them because '[mine] are the best ever.' As I was dropping the dough onto the cookie sheet I had an epiphany. I told my husband he could bake as many as he wanted, and I wrapped up the rest of the raw dough and brought it in to my co-workers with baking instructions. YOU GO GIRL!

"The hardest thing has been adjusting expectations as the weeks wore on. The first few weeks the weight dropped right off me. I was taking the initial weight loss, multiplying by the number of weeks until New Year's Eve, and eyeing a new cocktail dress. No such luck. Things ground to a halt after the eighth or ninth week, with only modest losses. But I'm still down 16 pounds and have either lost a minimal amount or not gained during the holiday season . . . Rick, thank you for choosing me to be in the group and for your and Ruth's tremendous support during this part of the voyage."

From Kathy, who lost 29 pounds and a total of 19 inches from her waist and hips:

"What have I learned over the past thirteen weeks? An enormous amount about myself: that I can say NO and mean it, that I can socialize and do okay, that having someone else to share the journey with makes all the difference in the world, that it feels good to accomplish some-thing and see the results beginning to change your thinking and actions, that there is a lot of bad information out there about food and diet that I spent years following and being frustrated with, that I don't have to be hungry or feel like I am being deprived, that I look forward to the weekly weigh-in with positive anticipation rather than negative fear, that whatever happened in childhood is no excuse for being overweight now—what's done is done, forget it, move on! Thank you for opening my eyes to all of this and my mind to accepting it."

From Pat, who lost 16 pounds:

"I am proud of myself this week as I have not only lost more inches, but I am down another pound . . . What really matters is that the weight continues to drop and I am bound and determined to reach my goal of 140 pounds . . . As for what tips I can provide, I always ask myself when I think I'm starving, 'Am I hungry, thirsty or tired?' Also when I am really wanting those red-light foods, I say to myself, 'Do I really need them or want them?' This gets me back on track. I also think about the end result and how I will look and feel. I know that summer is only months away and I want to look fine.

"When people comment on my weight loss and ask what diet I am on, I inform them this is my new way of eating. I have changed my lifestyle to improve my overall health . . . I keep using the red leather jacket as motivation. I try it on every Sunday morning to see the progress I have made, and it helps me to stay motivated."

From Nancy, who lost 13 pounds and over 10 inches from her waist and hips:

"Gosh, sometimes this is such a MENTAL struggle! Like many people, I've used food as a source of comfort over the years, particularly sweets. I spent two days in the hospital this week (asthma), so I felt sorry for myself and let myself eat things I know better than to eat — what's up with THAT? It's so frustrating.

"I think it's a mindset thing, in that I need to get back to the place where I simply choose not to eat sweets, where it's not even an option, let alone a desire. Does that make sense? I've reached that place with fried foods, in that I physically cannot handle eating anything fried anymore. I want to reach that same place with sweets, though admittedly they've had a much stronger 'hold' over me than fried foods ever did.

"Ah well, it's a journey and I press on. Besides, I have to remember that not only am I working toward losing weight and regaining my physical health, but I'm also sorting through a lot of long-standing mental attitudes at the same time. It's all part of the long-term success, I think, in that I have to deal with ALL aspects of the weight gain, not just the physical."

Congratulations everyone!

Where to Go from Here

Whether you have reached your weight-loss target by now and are ready to start Phase II of the G.I. Diet (see Chapter 6), or still hve some way to go, I would like to offer you what the original participants were offered at the end of the first 13 weeks of the e-Clinic; a nine-month extension of the program, which includes a monthly e-letter. These monthly e-letters will cover issues such as:

- How to stay the course
- Anxiety and fear of failure
- Maintaining motivation
- Dealing with temptation
- 5 essentials to permanent weight loss

Whether they wished to maintain their weight, or still had more weight to lose, the original Clinic members found this extension of the basic 13-week program extremely valuable. If you'd like to receive these nine monthly e-letters and record your progress on an optional personal website diary, all you have to do is to register at www.gidietclinic.com.

An exclusive website will support you during these nine months through a special members' question-and-answer forum, where I will respond to major issues raised in participants' diaries. In addition, you will receive access to recipes and exclusive content not available anywhere else on-line.

Once you register at www.gidietclinic.com, you will receive the first e-letter immediately, as well as access to your personal diary should you wish to track your results. All of your personal information will be kept strictly confidential. Any use of your questions or comments on the website will refer only to your first name.

The e-Clinic is a great opportunity to continue your positive experience with the G.I. Diet. For those of you who do not intend to continue with the nine-month extension, I would be most grateful if you would forward to me your weekly results from the 13 weeks in this book. If this is too much trouble, then just send me your starting measurements and your Week 13 measurements. Simply go to www.gidietclinic.com and click on the link to submit your results through a simple form. Any comments you might have would also be greatly appreciated.

PART III

Reaching Your Weight-Loss Target

Phase II

Well, you've made it. Congratulations! You've hit your target weight, you're digging out clothes you thought you'd never get into again, and you're finally on good terms with your full-length mirror. I hope you are relishing the new you and making the most of your increased energy. Now that you've graduated from Phase I, you can ease up a bit on limiting portion and serving sizes, and start adding some yellow-light foods to your diet. The idea here is to get comfortable with your G.I. program; this is how you're going to eat for the rest of your life.

The best news for most of us in Phase II is about alcohol and chocolate. While both were considered red-light in the Preliminary Phase and Phase I because of their high calorie content and tendency to spike blood sugar levels, in Phase II, it's time to reintroduce those little pleasures.

Alcohol

Medical research indicates that red wine, which is rich in flavonoids, can help reduce your risk of heart disease and stroke. So, in Phase II, a glass of red wine is allowed with dinner. Just because one glass is beneficial, however, doesn't mean that two or three is even better for you. Immoderate drinking undoes any health benefits, and alcohol contains calories. One glass of wine (5 ounces maximum) provides the optimum benefit.

Apart from red wine, keep your consumption of alcohol to a minimum. I realize that this can be difficult, since drinking is so often a part of social occasions and celebrations. An occasional lapse won't do a lot of harm, but it's easy to get carried away. There are various strategies to combat the social pressure to drink: you can graciously accept that glass of wine or cocktail, raise it in a toast, take a sip, and then discreetly leave it on the nearest buffet table. Faced with a tray of vodka martinis and glasses of red wine, stick with the wine, which lasts longer. Ruth drinks spritzers (wine mixed with soda water) on special occasions. And if you add lots of ice to your spritzer, you can reduce the alcohol even further while still joining in the party spirit. Whatever strategy you choose, always try to eat some food with your drink, even if it has to be a forbidden piece of cheese. The fat will slow the absorption of the alcohol and minimize its impact. (Of course, better to gravitate to the vegetable tray, but an emergency canapé won't be the ruin of you.)

Chocolate

For many of us, living without chocolate is not living. The good news is that in Phase II, some chocolate—the right sort of chocolate in the right amount—is acceptable. You may have heard that chocolate, like red wine, contains natural elements that help keep the arteries clear—but that's probably not your main motive for eating it. Chocolate combines fat, sugar and cocoa, all three of which please the palate. But most chocolate contains too much saturated fat and sugar, which keeps it deep in the red-light zone. Chocolate with a high cocoa content (70 percent or more) delivers more chocolate intensity per ounce, which means that even a square or two is satisfying. A square or two can give chocoholics the fix they need.

Green-Light Servings

PHASE II

Chocolate (at least 70 percent cocoa)	2 squares
Red wine	One 5-ounce glass

Moderation Is Key

Phase II, I must warn you, is a bit of a danger zone, the stage when most diets go off the rails. Most people think that when they reach their weight-loss goal, they can just drop the diet and go back to their old eating habits. And frankly, when I take a close look at what many of these diets expect you to live on, I can understand why people can't stick to them for long.

The reality is that, with some modifications, the G.I. program is your diet for life. But this shouldn't be a hardship, because the G.I. Diet was designed to give you a huge range of healthy choices, so you won't feel hungry, bored or unsatisfied. By now, you will know how to navigate your green-light way through the supermarket, decipher food labels and cook the green-light way. You are likely not even tempted to revert to your old ways. If you should fall prey to a double cheeseburger, you will be dismayed at how heavy, sluggish and ungratified you feel afterward. You will be too attached to your new feeling of lightness and level of energy to abandon them.

Before we look at some of the new options open to you in Phase II, a word of caution: your body can now function on less food than it did before you started. Why? Because you're lighter now, so your body requires fewer calories. Also, your metabolism has become more efficient, and your body has learned to do more with fewer calories. Keeping these two developments in mind, add a few more calories in Phase II, but don't go berserk. Don't make any significant changes in your serving sizes, and remember to make yellow-light foods the exception rather than the rule. This way, you will keep the balance between the calories you're consuming and the calories you're expending—and that is the secret to maintaining your new weight.

As you modestly increase portions of foods that you particularly enjoy and include some yellow-light items as a treat, keep monitoring your weight weekly, and adjust your servings up or down until your weight stays stable. This may take a few weeks of experimentation, but when you've reached the magic balance and can stay there comfortably, that's the formula for the rest of your days.

Here are some ideas of how you might alter the way you eat in Phase II.

Breakfast

- Increase cereal serving size from $^1/_2$ to $^2/_3$ of a cup.
- Add a slice of 100% whole-grain toast and a pat of margarine.
- Double the amount of sliced almonds on your cereal.
- Enjoy an extra slice of back bacon.
- Have a glass of unsweetened juice now and then.
- Add one of the yellow-light fruits—a banana or apricot—to your cereal.
- Go caffeinated in the coffee department, if you like, but try to keep it to one cup a day.

Lunch

I suggest you continue to eat lunch as you did in Phase I, as this is the one meal that already contained some compromises in the weight-loss portion of the program.

Dinner

- Add another boiled new potato.
- Increase the pasta serving from $^3/_4$ cup to 1 cup.
- As a special treat, have a 6-ounce steak instead of a 4-ounce one.
- Eat a few more olives and nuts—but only a few!
- Try a cob of sweet corn with a dab of margarine.
- Add a slice of high-fibre bread or crispbread.
- Enjoy a yellow-light cut of lamb or pork.

Snacks

- Have a maximum of 2 cups of air-popped popcorn.
- Increase your serving size of nuts to 10 or 12.
- Enjoy a square or two of 70 percent dark chocolate.
- Have a banana.
- Indulge in a scoop of low-fat ice cream or frozen yogurt.

Of course, Phase II is not, and shouldn't be, a straitjacket. If you live 90 percent within the guidelines of the diet, you are doing well. The idea that certain foods are completely and forever forbidden would drive you, sooner or later, back into their clutches. With the G.I. Diet, you are in control of what you eat, and that includes (with discipline, moderation and common sense) almost everything.

TO SUM UP
- In Phase II, use moderation and common sense in adjusting portions and servings.
- Don't view Phase II as a straitjacket. Occasional lapses are fine.

PART IV

The Recipes

Breakfast

HOMEY OATMEAL

This hot breakfast is guaranteed to keep you feeling satisfied all morning. You can vary the flavour by topping it with fresh fruit such as berries or chopped apple.

2 cups	skim milk
1 1/2 cups	water
3/4 tsp	ground cinnamon
1/2 tsp	salt
1 1/3 cups	large-flake oats
1/4 cup	wheat germ
1/4 cup	chopped almonds
3 tbsp	Splenda

1. In large pot, bring milk, water, cinnamon and salt to boil. Stir in oats and wheat germ and return to boil. Reduce heat to low and cook, stirring, for about 8 minutes or until thickened. Stir in almonds and Splenda.

Makes 4 servings.

HOMEMADE MUESLI

This cereal makes a delicious and healthy start to the day. Be sure to prepare it the night before so that it's ready to enjoy in the morning. Combine ⅓ cup of the Muesli with ⅓ cup of skim milk or water, and cover and refrigerate overnight. Then, in the morning, combine the mixture with 1 container (175 g) of non-fat, sugar-free fruit yogurt and enjoy it cold, or pop it in the microwave for a hot breakfast.

2 cups	large-flake oats
¾ cup	oat bran
¾ cup	sliced almonds
½ cup	shelled unsalted sunflower seeds
2 tbsp	wheat germ
¼ tsp	ground cinnamon

1. In large resealable plastic bag, combine oats, oat bran, almonds, sunflower seeds, wheat germ and cinnamon. Using rolling pin, crush mixture into coarse crumbs. Shake bag to combine mixture.

Makes 3 cups.

CINNAMON FRENCH TOAST

Serve this family favourite with slices of ham or back bacon and extra strawberries for a complete breakfast.

3/4 cup	liquid egg
1/2 cup	skim milk
1 tbsp	Splenda
1 tsp	vanilla
1/2 tsp	ground cinnamon
Pinch	salt
4	slices stone-ground whole wheat bread
1 tsp	canola oil
2 cups	sliced strawberries
1/2 cup	non-fat sugar-free fruit-flavoured yogurt

1. In shallow dish, whisk together liquid egg, milk, Splenda, vanilla, cinnamon and salt. Dip each slice of bread into egg mixture, making sure to coat both sides.

2. Meanwhile, brush oil onto non-stick griddle or large non-stick frying pan over medium-high heat. Cook for about 4 minutes, turning once, or until golden brown. Serve with strawberries and yogurt.

Makes 2 servings.

OATMEAL BUTTERMILK PANCAKES

Make pancake breakfasts a weekend tradition. Serve them with fresh fruit or applesauce.

3/4 cup	large-flake oats
2 cups	buttermilk
1 cup	whole wheat flour
1/4 cup	ground flaxseed
1 tbsp	Splenda
1 tsp	ground cinnamon
1 tsp	baking soda
1 tsp	baking powder
1/4 tsp	salt
1/2 cup	liquid egg
2 tbsp	canola oil
1 tsp	vanilla

1. In bowl, soak oats in buttermilk for 20 minutes.

2. In large bowl, combine flour, flaxseed, Splenda, cinnamon, baking soda, baking powder and salt.

3. In another bowl, whisk together liquid egg, oil and vanilla. Stir in soaked oats and buttermilk. Pour over flour mixture and stir until just mixed.

4. Meanwhile, heat non-stick griddle or large non-stick frying pan over medium heat. Ladle about 1/4 cup batter onto griddle for each pancake. Cook until bubbles appear on top, about 2 minutes.

5. Flip pancakes and cook for another 2 minutes or until golden. Transfer to plate and cover to keep warm. Repeat with remaining batter.

Makes 16 pancakes, 4 to 6 servings.

MINI BREAKFAST PUFFS

Ideal for rushed mornings, these muffin-sized puffs are packed with nutrition.

1 tsp	canola oil
¼ cup	diced onion
1	red pepper, diced
1 cup	chopped broccoli
1 ½ tsp	fresh thyme
¼ tsp	each salt and freshly ground pepper
¾ cup	crumbled light feta cheese
1 ½ cups	liquid egg
1 cup	skim milk
¼ cup	wheat bran
¼ cup	whole wheat flour

1. Preheat oven to 400°F.
2. In non-stick frying pan, heat oil over medium heat. Cook onion and red pepper for about 5 minutes or until softened. Add broccoli, thyme, salt and pepper; cover and steam for about 3 minutes or until broccoli is tender-crisp and bright green. Divide mixture among 12 greased muffin tins.
3. Sprinkle cheese over top of vegetable mixture in each cup.
4. In bowl, whisk together liquid egg, milk, bran and whole wheat flour. Divide evenly over vegetable mixture. Bake for about 20 minutes or until golden, set and puffed. Let cool slightly before serving.

Makes 12 puffs, 6 to 8 servings.

BACK BACON OMELETTE

The smoky flavour of bacon makes this omelette a hit. Serve this with fresh fruit and yogurt for a hearty breakfast.

1 tsp	canola oil
½ cup	liquid egg
1 tbsp	chopped fresh basil
1 tbsp	grated Parmesan cheese
Pinch	freshly ground pepper
2	slices back bacon or ham, chopped
¼	red or green pepper, chopped

1. In small non-stick frying pan, heat oil over medium-high heat. In bowl, using fork, stir together liquid egg, basil, cheese and pepper. Pour into frying pan and cook for about 5 minutes, lifting edges to allow uncooked egg to run underneath, until almost set.

2. Sprinkle bacon and red or green pepper over half of the omelette. Using spatula, fold over other half and cook for 1 minute.

Makes 1 serving.

ITALIAN OMELETTE

Omelettes are easy to make, and you can vary them by adding any number of fresh vegetables, a little cheese and/or some meat.

1 tsp	canola oil
½ cup	sliced mushrooms
½ cup	liquid egg
½ cup	tomato purée
1 tbsp	chopped fresh basil or oregano
1 oz	part-skim mozzarella cheese, shredded
Pinch	freshly ground pepper

1. In small non-stick frying pan, heat oil over medium-high heat. Add the mushrooms and sauté until tender, about 5 minutes. Transfer mushrooms to a plate and cover to keep warm.

2. In bowl, using fork, stir together liquid egg, tomato purée, basil, cheese and pepper. Pour into frying pan and cook for about 5 minutes, lifting edges to allow uncooked egg to run underneath, until almost set.

3. Sprinkle sautéed mushrooms over half of the omelette. Using spatula, fold over other half and cook for 1 minute.

Makes 1 serving.

VEGETARIAN OMELETTE

1 tsp	canola oil
1 cup	broccoli florets
½ cup	sliced mushrooms
½ cup	chopped red and green pepper
½ cup	liquid egg
1 oz	low-fat cheddar cheese, shredded
Pinch	freshly ground pepper

1. In small non-stick frying pan, heat oil over medium-high heat. Add the broccoli, mushrooms and pepper, and sauté until tender, about 5 minutes. Transfer vegetables to a plate and cover to keep warm.

2. In bowl, using fork, stir together liquid egg, cheese and pepper. Pour into frying pan and cook for about 5 minutes, lifting edges to allow uncooked egg to run underneath, until almost set.

3. Sprinkle sautéed vegetables over half of the omelette. Using spatula, fold over other half and cook for 1 minute.

Makes 1 serving.

WESTERN OMELETTE

1 tsp	canola oil
1 cup	chopped red and green pepper
1	small onion, chopped
½ cup	liquid egg
2	slices back bacon, lean deli ham or turkey breast, chopped
Pinch	red pepper flakes or cayenne pepper

1. In small non-stick frying pan, heat oil over medium-high heat. Add the pepper and onion, and sauté until tender, about 5 minutes. Transfer vegetables to a plate and cover to keep warm.

2. In bowl, using fork, stir together liquid egg, back bacon and red pepper flakes. Pour into frying pan and cook for about 5 minutes, lifting edges to allow uncooked egg to run underneath, until almost set.

3. Sprinkle sautéed vegetables over half of the omelette. Using spatula, fold over other half and cook for 1 minute.

Makes 1 serving.

Soups

MINESTRONE SOUP

This soup is one of my favourites because it contains both pasta and spinach. Serve it with a sprinkling of grated Parmesan cheese for extra flavour and a few more red pepper flakes to get your blood pumping.

2 tsp	canola oil
3	slices back bacon, chopped
1	onion, chopped
4	cloves garlic, minced
2	carrots, chopped
1	stalk celery, chopped
1 tbsp	dried oregano
1/2 tsp	red pepper flakes
1/4 tsp	each salt and freshly ground pepper
1	can (796 mL) plum tomatoes
6 cups	chicken stock (low-fat, low-sodium)
1	bag (300 g) baby spinach
1	can (540 mL) each red kidney beans and chickpeas, drained and rinsed
3/4 cup	ditali or tubetti pasta
1/3 cup	chopped fresh flat-leaf parsley
2 tbsp	chopped fresh basil (optional)

1. In large soup pot, heat oil over medium-high heat and cook back bacon for 2 minutes. Reduce heat to medium and add onion, garlic, carrots, celery, oregano, red pepper flakes, salt and pepper. Cook for about 10 minutes or until vegetables are softened and lightly browned.

2. Add tomatoes and crush using potato masher in pot. Pour in chicken stock; bring to boil. Reduce heat to simmer and add spinach, beans, chickpeas and pasta. Simmer for about 20 minutes or until pasta is tender. Stir in parsley and basil (if using).

Makes 6 servings.

TUSCAN WHITE BEAN SOUP

Serve this soup in deep Italian ceramic soup bowls and dream you're in Tuscany.

1 tbsp	extra-virgin olive oil
1	onion, chopped
4	cloves garlic, minced
1	carrot, chopped
1	stalk celery, chopped
4	fresh sage leaves or ½ tsp dried
6 cups	vegetable or chicken stock (low-fat, low-sodium)
2	cans (540 mL each) cannellini or white kidney beans, drained and rinsed
4 cups	shredded kale
Pinch	each salt and freshly ground pepper

1. In large soup pot, heat oil over medium heat. Add onion, garlic, carrot, celery and sage and cook for 5 minutes or until softened.

2. Add stock, beans, kale, salt and pepper, and cook, stirring occasionally, for about 20 minutes or until kale is tender.

Makes 4 servings.

QUICK AND EASY CHICKEN NOODLE SOUP

Why buy canned soup when you can make this simple homemade version?

2 tsp	extra-virgin olive oil
2	carrots, chopped
2	stalks celery, chopped
3	cloves garlic, chopped
1	onion, chopped
1 tbsp	chopped fresh thyme
6 cups	chicken stock (low-fat, low-sodium)
3	boneless skinless chicken breasts (4 oz each), diced
1 cup	frozen peas
3/4 cup	small pasta (such as ditali or tubetti)
1/4 cup	chopped fresh flat-leaf parsley
1/4 tsp	each salt and freshly ground pepper

1. In large soup pot, heat oil over medium-high heat. Add carrots, celery, garlic, onion and thyme, and cook for 10 minutes or until vegetables are slightly softened.

2. Pour in stock and bring to boil. Reduce heat to simmer and add chicken, peas and pasta. Simmer for 15 minutes or until chicken is no longer pink inside and pasta is al dente. Stir in parsley, salt, pepper.

Makes 6 servings.

HAM AND LENTIL SOUP

Canned lentils make this soup quick and easy to prepare, so keep some on hand. If you want to make this soup even more green-light, use dried lentils (see instructions at the bottom of this page).

1 tbsp	canola oil
1	onion, chopped
½ cup	diced celery
2	cloves garlic, minced
6 cups	chicken stock (low-fat, low-sodium)
2	cans (540 mL each) lentils, drained and rinsed
6 oz	black forest ham, diced
1	red pepper, diced
2	tomatoes, seeded and diced
2 tbsp	chopped flat-leaf parsley

1. In large soup pot, heat oil over medium heat. Add onion, celery and garlic, and cook for about 5 minutes or until softened. Add stock, lentils, ham and red pepper; bring to boil. Reduce heat and add tomatoes. Cover and simmer for 20 minutes. Stir in parsley.

Makes 4 servings.

Variation:

Use 1 cup dried green or brown lentils. Add with stock, and cover and simmer for about 30 minutes or until tender.

Salads

RAITA SALAD

This recipe is based on the refreshing Indian condiment. Try serving this salad with Chicken Curry (see recipe, page 252).

1	bag (300 g) baby spinach
1	medium English cucumber, quartered lengthwise and sliced into 1/2-inch chunks
2	tomatoes, chopped
1/2	red onion, thinly sliced
1 cup	low-fat plain yogurt
1/2 tsp	ground cumin
1/4 tsp	salt

1. In large bowl, toss together spinach, cucumber, tomatoes and red onion.
2. In another bowl, stir together yogurt, cumin and salt. Add to spinach mixture and toss to coat.

Makes 4 servings.

TANGY RED AND GREEN COLESLAW

Using a vinaigrette in coleslaw makes it low-fat and really tangy! This is a great keeper salad for the refrigerator or to tote along to a potluck.

4 cups	finely shredded green cabbage
2 cups	finely shredded red cabbage
2	carrots, shredded
1/2 cup	thinly sliced celery
1/4 cup	chopped fresh flat-leaf parsley
1/2 cup	cider vinegar
2 tbsp	canola oil
2 tsp	Splenda
1 tsp	celery seeds
1/2 tsp	salt
Pinch	freshly ground pepper

1. In large bowl, toss together green and red cabbage, carrots, celery and parsley.
2. In small bowl, whisk together vinegar, oil, Splenda, celery seeds, salt and pepper. Pour over cabbage mixture and toss to coat.

Makes 4 to 6 servings.

BASIC G.I. SALAD

1 ½ cups	lettuce (such as arugula, baby spinach, Boston, iceberg, leaf, mesclun, romaine or watercress), torn or coarsely chopped
1	small carrot, grated
½	red, yellow or green pepper, diced
1	plum tomato, cut into wedges
½ cup	sliced cucumber
¼ cup	chopped red onion (optional)

Basic G.I. Vinaigrette:

1 tbsp	vinegar (such as balsamic, cider, red wine, rice or white wine) or lemon juice
1 tsp	extra-virgin olive oil or canola oil
½ tsp	Dijon mustard
1	clove garlic, crushed (optional)
Pinch	each salt and freshly ground pepper
Pinch	finely chopped fresh herb of choice (such as basil, marjoram, mint, oregano or thyme)

1. In large bowl, toss together lettuce, carrot, pepper, tomato, cucumber and onion.
2. Vinaigrette: In small bowl, whisk together vinegar, oil, mustard, garlic, salt, pepper and herb.
3. Pour vinaigrette over greens and toss to coat.

Makes 1 serving.

Variations:

To make a meal out of this salad, add some protein with 4 oz canned tuna, cooked salmon, tofu, kidney beans, chickpeas, cooked chicken or another lean meat.

Make Ahead: Both the salad and the dressing can be prepared ahead and stored separately, covered, for about 2 days.

CAESAR SALAD

We all need a Caesar salad in our recipe repertoire. No one will guess that tahini is the secret ingredient that makes this green-light version every bit as creamy as Chef Caesar Cardini's original.

3	slices whole-grain bread
2 tsp	extra-virgin olive oil
Pinch	each salt and freshly ground pepper
1	large head romaine lettuce

Dressing:

3	cloves garlic, minced
3	anchovy fillets, finely minced
2 tbsp	tahini
1 tsp	Dijon mustard
1/2 tsp	Worcestershire sauce
1/2 tsp	each salt and freshly ground pepper
3 tbsp	fresh lemon juice
2 tbsp	warm water
1 1/2 tbsp	extra-virgin olive oil

1. Preheat oven to 350°F.
2. Cut bread into 1/2-inch pieces and place in bowl. Add oil, salt and pepper and toss to coat well. Arrange in single layer on rimmed baking sheet. Bake for 20 minutes or until golden and crisp. Let cool.
3. Wash lettuce and tear into bite-size pieces; place in large bowl.
4. **Dressing:** In small bowl, stir together garlic, anchovies, tahini, mustard, Worcestershire sauce, salt and pepper. Whisk in lemon juice, water and oil.
5. Pour dressing over lettuce and toss to coat. Sprinkle with croutons.

Makes 4 servings.

GREEK SALAD

2 cups	torn iceberg lettuce
1/2	cucumber, chopped
2	tomatoes, chopped
6	kalamata olives
1/2	red onion, sliced
1/4 cup	crumbled light feta cheese
1 tbsp	red wine vinegar
2 tsp	extra-virgin olive oil
1 tsp	fresh lemon juice
3/4 tsp	dried oregano
Pinch	each salt and freshly ground pepper

1. In bowl, toss together lettuce, cucumber, tomatoes, olives, red onion, and crumbled feta.

2. In small bowl, whisk together vinegar, oil, lemon juice, oregano, salt and pepper. Pour over lettuce and toss to coat.

Makes 2 servings.

COLD NOODLE SALAD WITH CUCUMBER AND SESAME

These refreshing noodles pair well with Ginger-Wasabi Halibut (see recipe, page 252).

6 oz	thin pasta (vermicelli, capellini or spaghettini)
1 tbsp	rice vinegar
4 tsp	Splenda
2 tsp	soy sauce
1/2	English cucumber, quartered lengthwise and thinly sliced
2 tbsp	toasted sesame seeds

1. In large pot of boiling salted water, cook pasta until al dente, about 4 minutes. Drain and rinse under cold water. Place in large bowl.

2. In small bowl, stir together vinegar, Splenda and soy sauce. Pour over cooked noodles, and stir in cucumber and sesame seeds; toss well to coat.

Makes 6 servings.

G.I. PASTA SALAD

½ to ¾ cup	cooked whole wheat pasta (spirals, shells or similar size)
1 cup	chopped cooked vegetables (such as broccoli, asparagus, peppers or green onions)
¼ cup	light tomato sauce or other low-fat or non-fat pasta sauce
4 oz	cooked chicken or other lean meat, such as lean ground turkey or lean chicken sausage, chopped

1. Place the pasta, vegetables, tomato sauce and chicken in a bowl and stir to mix well. Refrigerate, covered, until ready to use, then heat in the microwave or serve chilled.

Makes 1 serving.

Variation:

You can use the proportions here as a guide and vary the vegetables, sauce and source of protein to suit your tastes and add variety to your pasta salads.

TABBOULEH SALAD

You often see this salad in the grocery store deli, but it's very simple to make at home. The chickpeas add more fibre.

1 ½ cups	water
3/4 cup	bulgur
½ tsp	grated lemon zest
2 tbsp	fresh lemon juice
2 tbsp	extra-virgin olive oil
1	small clove garlic, minced
½ tsp	each salt and freshly ground pepper
¼ tsp	ground cumin
1	can (540 mL) chickpeas, drained and rinsed
3	plum tomatoes, diced
¼	cucumber, diced
1 cup	finely chopped fresh flat-leaf parsley
½ cup	finely chopped fresh mint
1 tbsp	chopped fresh chives

1. In saucepan, bring water to boil; add bulgur. Cover, reduce heat to low and cook for about 10 minutes or until water is absorbed. Using fork, scrape into large bowl; let cool.

2. In small bowl, whisk together lemon zest and juice, oil, garlic, salt, pepper and cumin; pour over bulgur. Stir in chickpeas, tomatoes, cucumber, parsley, mint and chives until well combined.

Makes 4 to 6 servings.

Make Ahead: This salad will last up to 3 days in the refrigerator.

MIXED BEAN SALAD

1	can (540 mL) mixed beans, drained and rinsed
1/2	cucumber, chopped
1	tomato, chopped
1 cup	cooked whole wheat pasta (small shells, macaroni or similar size)
2 tbsp	chopped fresh flat-leaf parsley
1 tbsp	red wine vinegar
2 tsp	extra-virgin olive oil
1/4 tsp	Dijon mustard
Pinch	each salt and freshly ground pepper
Pinch	finely chopped fresh herbs (such as thyme or oregano)

1. Place beans in large bowl and add cucumber, tomato, pasta and parsley.
2. In small bowl, whisk together vinegar, oil, mustard, salt, pepper and herbs. Pour over salad and toss to coat.

Makes 2 servings.

WALDORF CHICKEN AND RICE SALAD

3/4 cup	cooked basmati or brown rice
1	medium apple, chopped
1 or 2	stalks celery, chopped
1/4 cup	walnuts
4 oz	cooked chicken, chopped
1 tbsp	store-bought light buttermilk dressing

1. Place rice, apple, celery, walnuts and chicken in large bowl. Pour in buttermilk dressing and stir to mix.

Makes 1 serving.

CRAB SALAD IN TOMATO SHELLS

Beefsteak tomatoes are ideal for this dish because their large size will accommodate the filling, and pulp and seeds are easy to scoop out.

2	packages (200 g each) frozen crab, thawed
4	large beefsteak tomatoes
¼ cup	fat-free mayonnaise
2 tbsp	low-fat sour cream
½ tsp	grated lemon zest
1 tbsp	fresh lemon juice
2 tsp	chopped fresh tarragon
Pinch	each salt and freshly ground pepper
1 cup	coarsely chopped cooked chickpeas
½	red pepper, diced
¼ cup	finely diced celery
¼ cup	chopped fresh flat-leaf parsley
2 tbsp	chopped fresh chives
2 tbsp	shredded carrot

1. Place crab in fine-mesh sieve; press out any liquid. Remove and discard any cartilage if necessary; set aside crab.

2. Cut top quarter off tomatoes. Using small spoon, scoop out seeds and pulp. Place tomatoes cut side down on paper towel–lined plate.

3. In large bowl, stir together mayonnaise, sour cream, lemon zest and juice, tarragon, salt and pepper. Add chickpeas, red pepper, celery, parsley, chives and carrot. Add crab and stir to combine. Divide crab mixture among tomatoes.

Makes 4 servings.

Meatless

FETTUCCINE PRIMAVERA

Primavera means "springtime" in Italian, and you can use your favourite spring vegetables, such as asparagus or fiddleheads, in this pasta. Fortunately, you can get peppers, tomatoes and peas year-round, so you can make this dish any time.

¼ cup	extra-virgin olive oil
2 cups	cubed firm tofu
3	cloves garlic, minced
¼ tsp	red pepper flakes
½ cup	vegetable cocktail juice
2 cups	chopped fresh asparagus or peas
1	red pepper, thinly sliced
1	carrot, thinly sliced
1	yellow zucchini, thinly sliced
6 oz	whole wheat fettuccine or linguine pasta
2	plum tomatoes, chopped
¼ cup	chopped fresh flat-leaf parsley
2 tbsp	grated Parmesan cheese

1. In non-stick frying pan, heat 2 tbsp of the oil over medium-high heat. Brown tofu on all sides for about 2 minutes; remove to plate. Reserve oil.

2. In large shallow saucepan, heat remaining oil and reserved oil over medium heat. Cook garlic and red pepper flakes for 1 minute. Add vegetable cocktail juice; bring to boil. Reduce heat and simmer for 1 minute. Add asparagus, red pepper, carrot and zucchini; cook, stirring, for 10 minutes or until vegetables are tender-crisp.

3. Meanwhile, in large pot of boiling salted water, cook fettuccine for 8 minutes or until al dente. Drain and return to pot. Add vegetables and tofu, and toss to coat. Stir in tomatoes, parsley and Parmesan cheese.

Makes 4 servings.

BARLEY RISOTTO WITH LEEKS, LEMON AND PEAS

Unlike traditional risotto, this barley version doesn't need to be watched or stirred continuously.

1 tbsp	extra-virgin olive oil
½ cup	chopped leek (white and light green parts only)
2	cloves garlic, minced
½ tsp	chopped fresh thyme
1 cup	barley
¼ cup	dry white wine or vermouth
3 cups	chicken stock (low-fat, low-sodium) (and up to ½ cup more if needed)
1 cup	fresh or thawed frozen peas
	Zest and juice of 1 medium lemon
2 tbsp	grated Parmesan cheese
¼ tsp	each salt and freshly ground pepper

1. In saucepan, heat oil over medium-high heat; cook leek, garlic and thyme, stirring, for 3 minutes or until softened. Stir in barley until well coated.

2. Add wine and stir until absorbed. Add stock and bring to boil. Cover and reduce heat to low; simmer, stirring occasionally, for 40 to 45 minutes or until barley is tender. If necessary, stir in a little more stock or hot water near the end of cooking time to maintain a creamy consistency. Stir in peas, lemon zest and juice, and Parmesan cheese; season with salt and pepper.

Makes 4 to 6 servings.

VEGETABLE CRUMBLE

We usually think of a crumble as dessert, but this one makes a delicious vegetarian main dish, or a side dish for meat or fish.

1 tbsp	extra-virgin olive oil
1 cup	sliced leeks (white and light green parts only)
1	onion, chopped
1	zucchini, cut into 1-inch pieces (about 1 cup)
1	large carrot, cut into 1-inch pieces (about 1 cup)
1	sweet potato, peeled and cut into 1-inch pieces (about 1 cup)
4 oz	mushrooms, quartered
1	stalk celery, sliced into ½-inch pieces (about ¾ cup)
½	red pepper, cut into 1-inch pieces
1 tbsp	chopped fresh thyme
¼ cup	whole wheat flour
1 cup	drained canned plum tomatoes, roughly chopped
1 cup	vegetable stock (low-fat, low-sodium)
½ cup	skim milk
¼ cup	chopped fresh flat-leaf parsley
½ tsp	each salt and freshly ground pepper

Topping:

¼ cup	non-hydrogenated soft margarine
¼ cup	whole wheat flour
¼ cup	wheat bran
¾ cup	shredded low-fat cheddar cheese
½ cup	chopped mixed nuts
2 tbsp	sesame seeds

1. Preheat oven to 375°F.

2. In large saucepan, heat oil over medium-high heat. Cook leeks and onion for 5 minutes or until softened. Add zucchini, carrot, sweet potato, mushrooms, celery, red pepper and thyme. Cook, stirring often, for 10 minutes. Stir in flour; cook for 1 minute.

3. Stir in tomatoes, stock, milk, parsley, salt and pepper; bring to boil. Reduce heat, cover and simmer for about 15 minutes or until vegetables are tender.

4. **Topping:** Meanwhile, in bowl, combine margarine, flour and bran. Using your fingers, rub ingredients together until mixture is crumbly. Stir in cheese, nuts and sesame seeds.

5. Spoon vegetable mixture into 8-cup shallow baking dish. Sprinkle topping over top, distributing evenly.

6. Bake for 30 minutes or until topping is crisp and golden, and vegetable mixture is bubbling.

Makes 4 to 6 servings.

Make Ahead: Add 2 tbsp whole wheat flour to filling in Step 2. After Step 5, wrap well and freeze up to 1 month. Bake from frozen, increasing cooking time by 30 to 45 minutes.

BEAN AND ONION PIZZA

Here's a restaurant favourite for your G.I. lifestyle.

Pizza Dough:

3/4 cup	warm water
2 1/4 tsp	active dry yeast
1 1/3 cups	whole wheat flour
1/2 cup	wheat bran
Pinch	salt

Topping:

1 tsp	canola oil
2	onions, thinly sliced
2	cloves garlic, minced
3/4 tsp	finely chopped fresh thyme
Pinch	each salt and freshly ground pepper
1/4 cup	sun-dried tomatoes
1/2 cup	boiling water
1 cup	cooked red kidney beans
3/4 cup	low-fat pasta sauce
2 tbsp	chopped fresh basil
3/4 cup	crumbled light feta cheese

1. Pizza Dough: Pour water into large bowl and sprinkle with yeast. Let stand for about 10 minutes or until frothy. Stir in 1 1/4 cups of the flour, the bran and salt until a ragged dough forms. Let stand, covered, for 30 minutes. Place dough on a floured surface and knead, adding more of the remaining flour as necessary, just until it forms a soft, slightly sticky dough. Place in a greased bowl, cover and let rest until doubled in bulk, about 1 hour.

2. Topping: In non-stick frying pan, heat oil over medium-high heat. Cook onions and garlic, stirring, until onions start to become golden, about 3 minutes. Reduce heat to medium and add thyme, salt and pepper. Continue cooking, stirring occasionally, until onions are soft and golden brown, about 15 minutes.

3. Soak sun-dried tomatoes in boiling water for 5 minutes. Drain and discard water, and chop tomatoes.

4. Preheat oven to 425°F.

5. Punch down dough and roll out on a floured surface to fit a 12- or 14-inch round pizza pan. Place dough on pan, stretching as necessary to fit.

6. Place beans in large mixing bowl and mash, using a potato masher. Stir in pasta sauce, sun-dried tomatoes and basil. Spread topping over pizza dough. Top with sautéed onions, and sprinkle with feta.

7. Bake for about 20 minutes or until golden and crisp.

Makes 4 servings.

EASY-BAKE LASAGNA

Though cooking the G.I. way usually means starting from scratch, there are some handy convenience products that are green-light, such as pasta sauce! This lasagna is great for a crowd. Just add a tossed salad.

12	whole wheat lasagna noodles
2 tsp	canola oil
1	onion, chopped
1	red pepper, chopped
8 oz	mushrooms, sliced
1/4 tsp	each salt and freshly ground pepper
1	bag (300 g) baby spinach
1 1/2 cups	diced firm tofu
1 cup	1% cottage cheese
1/3 cup	liquid egg
1	jar (700 mL) low-fat pasta sauce
1 1/2 cups	shredded part-skim mozzarella cheese
2 tbsp	grated Parmesan cheese

1. Preheat oven to 350°F

2. In large pot of boiling salted water, cook lasagna noodles for about 10 minutes or until al dente. Drain and rinse under cold water. Lay noodles flat on damp tea towels; set aside.

3. Meanwhile, in large non-stick frying pan, heat oil over medium-high heat. Cook onion, red pepper, mushrooms, salt and pepper for about 8 minutes, or until golden brown and liquid evaporates. Add spinach and cook, stirring, for 2 minutes or until wilted. Stir in tofu.

4. In small bowl, stir together cottage cheese and liquid egg; set aside.

5. Ladle 1/2 cup of the pasta sauce in the bottom of a 13- by 9-inch glass baking dish. Lay 3 noodles on top of sauce. Spread one-third of the spinach mixture over top, then one-third of the cottage cheese mixture. Spread with another 1/2 cup of the pasta sauce. Sprinkle with 1/3 cup of the mozzarella. Repeat layers,

ending with noodles on top. Spread with remaining sauce and sprinkle with remaining mozzarella and Parmesan cheese.

6. Cover with foil and bake for 45 minutes. Uncover and bake for 15 minutes or until bubbly and knife inserted in centre is hot to the touch. Let cool 10 minutes before cutting and serving.

Makes 8 servings.

VEGETARIAN MOUSSAKA

Traditionally made with ground lamb, moussaka can be made green-light by using vegetables.

2	large eggplants (about 3 lbs total)
2 tsp	salt
1 tsp	canola oil
2	large onions, finely chopped
3	cloves garlic, minced
1	each red and green pepper, diced
1 tbsp	dried oregano
1 tsp	ground cinnamon
1/2 tsp	freshly ground pepper
1/4 tsp	ground allspice
1	can (796 mL) diced tomatoes
1/4 cup	tomato paste
1	can (540 mL) chickpeas, drained and rinsed
1/4 cup	chopped fresh flat-leaf parsley

Cheese Sauce:

2 tbsp	canola oil
1/4 cup	whole wheat flour
2 cups	warm skim milk
1/4 tsp	salt
Pinch	each ground nutmeg and freshly ground pepper
2/3 cup	liquid egg
1/2 cup	1% pressed cottage cheese
1 cup	crumbled light feta cheese

1. Preheat oven to 425°F.

2. Cut eggplants into $1/4$-inch-thick slices and layer in a colander, sprinkling each layer with some of the salt. Let stand for 30 minutes, then rinse slices

and drain well. Place on baking sheets lined with parchment paper and roast, in batches if necessary, for about 20 minutes or until tender. Set aside. Reduce oven temperature to 350°F.

3. In a large, shallow Dutch oven or deep non-stick frying pan, heat oil over medium heat. Cook onions, garlic, red and green peppers, oregano, cinnamon, pepper and allspice until onions have softened, about 5 minutes. Add tomatoes and tomato paste; bring to boil. Add chickpeas and parsley, reduce heat and simmer for 15 minutes.

4. Cheese Sauce: In a saucepan, heat oil over medium heat. Stir in flour and cook for 1 minute. Whisk in milk and cook, whisking gently, for about 10 minutes or until mixture is thick enough to coat the back of a spoon. Stir in salt, nutmeg and pepper. Let cool slightly and whisk in liquid egg and cottage cheese.

5. Spread one-third of the tomato sauce in the bottom of a 13- by 9-inch baking dish. Top with one-third of the eggplant slices and one-quarter of the feta cheese. Repeat the layers. After the last layer of eggplant, spread the cheese sauce evenly over the top and sprinkle with the remaining feta.

6. Bake for about 1 hour or until top is golden brown. Let stand for 10 minutes before serving.

Makes 8 servings.

Fish and Seafood

SALMON PASTA

When you can't get to the market for fresh salmon, use 2 cans of salmon or tuna instead.

2 tsp	canola oil
1	small onion, finely chopped
2	cloves garlic, minced
2 cups	chicken or fish stock (low-fat, low-sodium)
1 cup	whole wheat macaroni
1 1/2 cups	chopped broccoli
1/3 cup	light herb and garlic cream cheese
6 oz	skinless salmon fillet
2 tbsp	chopped fresh flat-leaf parsley
Pinch	each salt and freshly ground pepper

1. Preheat oven to 425°F.

2. In saucepan, heat 1 tsp of the oil over medium heat. Cook onion and garlic for about 3 minutes or until softened. Add stock and bring to boil. Add pasta and cover; reduce heat to simmer and cook for 10 minutes. Stir in broccoli and cream cheese. Remove from heat. Let stand, covered, for 10 minutes while salmon cooks.

3. Meanwhile, rub remaining oil over fillet and sprinkle with parsley, salt and pepper. Roast in small baking pan for about 10 minutes or until salmon is opaque and flakes easily with a fork. Break up salmon into chunks and add to pasta mixture. Stir gently to combine.

Makes 2 servings.

THAI RED CURRY SHRIMP PASTA

The combination of curry spices, lime and cilantro are hallmarks of Thai cooking.

1 lb	large raw shrimp, peeled and deveined
1 tsp	Thai red curry paste
1 tbsp	extra-virgin olive oil
4	cloves garlic, minced
2	large tomatoes, peeled, seeded and chopped
3/4 cup	dry white wine
	Zest and juice of 1 lime
1/4 tsp	each salt and freshly ground pepper
2 tbsp	chopped fresh cilantro
6 oz	whole wheat spaghettini or linguine
	Lime wedges

1. In bowl, toss shrimp with curry paste until well coated. Cover and refrigerate for at least 2 hours or up to 8 hours.

2. In large non-stick frying pan, heat oil over medium heat. Cook garlic just until starting to turn golden, 1 to 2 minutes. Add tomatoes, wine, lime zest and juice, salt and pepper; bring to boil. Reduce heat and simmer until sauce reduces and thickens, about 8 minutes. Add shrimp and cook, stirring, until pink and firm, 3 to 4 minutes. Stir in cilantro.

3. Meanwhile, in large pot of boiling salted water, cook pasta until al dente, about 8 minutes. Drain and add pasta to shrimp mixture. Toss to coat with sauce. Serve with lime wedges.

Makes 4 servings.

G.I. FISH FILLET

You can use virtually any fish in this simple recipe; salmon and trout are favourites in our house. This makes 1 serving, but you can multiply portions as necessary.

4 oz	fish fillet
1 to 2 tsp	fresh lemon juice
pinch	freshly ground pepper

1. Place fish fillet in microwave-safe dish and sprinkle with lemon juice and pepper. Cover dish with microwave-safe plastic wrap, folding back one corner slightly to allow steam to escape.

2. Microwave on High until fish is opaque and easily with a fork, 4 to 5 minutes. Let stand for 2 minutes, then serve.

Makes 1 serving.

CITRUS-POACHED HADDOCK

Citrus fruits and fish are made for each other. This simple dish is impressive enough for company.

1	small onion, finely chopped
1	clove garlic, minced
¼ cup	orange juice
¼ cup	dry white wine or vermouth
1 tsp	lemon zest
1 tbsp	fresh lemon juice
¼ cup	fish, chicken or vegetable stock (low-fat, low-sodium)
1 lb	haddock fillet, cut into 4 pieces
2 tbsp	chopped fresh flat-leaf parsley or dill
¼ tsp	each salt and freshly ground pepper

1. In large frying pan, bring onion, garlic, orange juice, wine, and lemon zest and juice to boil. Boil until onion is softened and liquid is reduced by half, about 5 minutes.

2. Add stock and return to boil. Place haddock in frying pan; reduce heat and simmer gently, covered, for 10 minutes or until fish is opaque and flakes easily with a fork. Using slotted spoon, remove haddock to platter and cover to keep warm.

3. Bring poaching liquid to boil and reduce by one-third. Stir in parsley and season with salt and pepper. Pour sauce over fish.

Makes 4 servings.

GINGER-WASABI HALIBUT

This fish can also be cooked on the barbecue. Serve it with Cold Noodle Salad with Cucumber and Sesame (see recipe, page 224) for a refreshing meal.

2 tbsp	Dijon mustard
2 tsp	wasabi powder
3 tbsp	mirin or sweet sherry
2 tbsp	minced ginger root
2 tbsp	chopped fresh cilantro
1 lb	halibut, cut into 4 pieces

1. Preheat oven to 350°F.

2. In bowl, stir together mustard and wasabi powder. Stir in mirin, ginger and cilantro. Place fish in marinade and turn to coat. Let stand at room temperature for 20 minutes.

3. Place halibut on baking sheet and bake for 8 to 10 minutes or until firm to the touch.

Makes 4 servings.

GRILLED TUNA WITH CHIMICHURRI SAUCE

Chimichurri is traditionally served with Argentinian barbecued beef (asado), but is also delicious with grilled tuna. This recipe makes extra sauce, which can be served with poultry or meat, or stirred into hot rice.

4	tuna steaks, about ½-inch thick (4 oz each)
½ tsp	each salt and freshly ground pepper

Chimichurri Sauce:

4	cloves garlic, minced
½	red onion, finely chopped
½	red pepper, finely chopped
¼ cup	chopped fresh cilantro
¼ cup	chopped fresh flat-leaf parsley
1 tbsp	chopped fresh oregano
½ cup	vegetable stock (low-fat, low-sodium)
2 tbsp	extra-virgin olive oil
2 tbsp	sherry or red wine vinegar
Pinch	each salt and freshly ground pepper

1. Preheat oiled grill to medium-high.

2. **Chimichurri Sauce:** In bowl, combine garlic, red onion, red pepper, cilantro, parsley and oregano. Stir in stock, oil, sherry, salt and pepper.

3. Season fish with salt and pepper, and grill until just charred on outside and rare in centre, about 2 minutes per side. Serve with a dollop of Chimichurri Sauce on top.

Makes 4 servings.

Make Ahead: Refrigerate sauce in airtight container up to 5 days.

PAN-SEARED WHITE FISH WITH MANDARIN SALSA

A quick, bright citrusy salsa lends a tropical note to this hearty fish fillet. You can use tilapia, haddock or catfish for this elegant meal.

Mandarin Salsa:

2	cans (284 mL each) no-sugar-added mandarin oranges, drained
1	red pepper, diced
½ cup	diced cucumber
¼ cup	finely diced red onion
3 tbsp	chopped fresh cilantro
1 tbsp	rice vinegar
¼ tsp	salt
Pinch	freshly ground pepper

Fish Fillets:

¾ cup	fresh whole wheat breadcrumbs
¼ cup	chopped fresh flat-leaf parsley
2 tbsp	wheat bran
2 tbsp	wheat germ
1 tbsp	chopped fresh tarragon
¼ tsp	salt
¼ tsp	freshly ground pepper
¼ cup	whole wheat flour
⅓ cup	liquid egg
4	white fish fillets (4 oz each)
4 tsp	canola oil

1. **Mandarin Salsa:** Coarsely chop mandarin slices and place in a bowl. Add red pepper, cucumber, onion, cilantro, vinegar, salt and pepper. Toss to combine.

2. **Fish Fillets:** Prepare three large, shallow dishes. In the first, combine bread crumbs, parsley, bran, wheat germ, tarragon, salt and pepper. In the second,

place the flour. In the third, place the liquid egg. Dredge a fish fillet with flour first, shaking off the excess. Coat with liquid egg, then dredge with breadcrumb mixture. Repeat with remaining fillets. Place prepared fillets on a plate lined with waxed paper and set aside.

3. In a large non-stick frying pan, heat half the oil over medium-high heat. Add 2 of the fillets and cook, turning once, until golden brown, about 10 minutes. Repeat with the remaining oil and fillets. Serve topped with Mandarin Salsa.

Makes 4 servings.

Poultry

CHICKEN FRIED RICE

Chinese fried rice is generally high in fat and low in protein and fibre. This low-G.I. version is loaded with chicken and colourful vegetables, and won't leave you feeling hungry again soon after eating it.

3/4 cup	brown rice
Pinch	salt
1 1/2 cups	chicken stock (low-fat, low-sodium)
1 tsp	sesame oil
2	boneless skinless chicken breasts (4 oz each), chopped
1 cup	sliced mushrooms
1	green onion, chopped
2	carrots, diced
1/2 cup	sliced celery
1 cup	cooked chickpeas
1/4 cup	light soy sauce
2 cups	bean sprouts

1. In saucepan, bring rice, salt and 1 1/4 cups of the chicken stock to boil. Reduce heat to low, cover and cook for about 25 minutes or until liquid is absorbed. Fluff with fork and set aside.

2. In large non-stick frying pan, heat oil over medium-high heat. Cook chicken and mushrooms for about 8 minutes or until chicken is no longer pink inside. Add green onion, carrots, celery, chickpeas and cooked rice. Cook, stirring, for 2 minutes to combine.

3. Add remaining chicken stock and soy sauce, and cook for 5 minutes. Add bean sprouts and toss to combine.

Makes 4 servings.

Variation: Substitute vegetable stock for the chicken stock, and 1/2 cup chopped extra-firm tofu for the chicken.

CHICKEN CURRY

	Vegetable oil cooking spray (preferably canola or olive oil)
1	medium onion, sliced
1 to 2 tbsp	curry powder (or more, to taste)
1 cup	sliced carrots
1 cup	chopped celery
1/2 cup	basmati rice
1	medium apple, chopped
1/4 cup	raisins
1	boneless skinless chicken breast (8 oz), cooked

1. Spray non-stick frying pan with oil, then place over medium heat. Add onion and curry powder, stir to coat onion with curry, then sauté for 1 minute.
2. Add carrots and celery, stir to mix, then sauté for 1 minute.
3. Add rice, apple, raisins and 1 cup of water, and stir to mix. Cover and let simmer until liquid is absorbed.
4. Add cooked chicken and heat through for 2 minutes.

Makes 2 servings.

CHICKEN SCHNITZEL

Kids love this dish. You can substitute more traditional veal scaloppine for the chicken.

4	boneless skinless chicken breasts (4 oz each)
1/2 cup	whole wheat flour
1/2 tsp	each salt and freshly ground pepper
2	omega-3 egg whites
1/2 cup	wheat bran
1/4 cup	wheat germ
1/4 cup	fine dry whole wheat breadcrumbs
1 tsp	grated orange zest
1 tbsp	extra-virgin olive oil
1/2 cup	fresh orange juice
1/2 cup	chicken stock (low-fat, low-sodium)
1/2 cup	thinly sliced dried apricots
1/4 cup	chopped green onion

1. Using meat mallet or rolling pin, pound chicken breasts between 2 pieces of plastic wrap until about 1/4 inch thick.

2. In large, shallow dish or pie plate, combine flour, salt and pepper. In another shallow dish or pie plate, whisk egg whites. In third dish or pie plate, combine bran, wheat germ, breadcrumbs and orange zest.

3. Pat chicken dry and dredge in flour mixture, shaking off excess. Dip in egg whites, letting excess drip off, then dredge in bran mixture, coating completely.

4. In large non-stick frying pan, heat oil over medium-high heat. Fry chicken (in batches, if necessary) for 4 minutes per side or until golden brown and just cooked through. Transfer schnitzel to platter and place in 200°F oven to keep warm.

5. In same frying pan, combine orange juice, stock and apricots. Bring to boil and reduce until slightly thickened and syrupy, about 3 minutes. Stir in green onion. Pour sauce over schnitzel.

Makes 4 servings.

CHICKEN JAMBALAYA

Jambalaya is a traditional Cajun dish in which rice is used to sop up the rich juices of the stew.

2 tsp	canola oil
2	stalks celery, chopped
2	cloves garlic, minced
1	onion, chopped
1 lb	boneless skinless chicken breasts, cut into ¹/₂-inch cubes
2 tsp	dried thyme
2 tsp	dried oregano
1 tsp	chili powder
¹/₄ tsp	cayenne pepper (optional)
2 cups	chicken stock (low-fat, low-sodium)
2	green peppers, diced
1	can (796 mL) stewed tomatoes
1	can (540 mL) kidney beans, drained and rinsed
³/₄ cup	brown rice
1	bay leaf
¹/₄ cup	chopped fresh flat-leaf parsley

1. In a Dutch oven, heat oil over medium-high heat. Cook celery, garlic and onion until onion has softened, about 5 minutes. Add chicken, thyme, oregano, chili powder and cayenne (if using) and cook, stirring, for 5 minutes.

2. Add stock, green peppers, tomatoes, kidney beans, rice and bay leaf, and bring to boil. Reduce heat to low, cover and simmer, stirring occasionally, for about 35 minutes or until rice is tender. Let stand for 5 minutes. Remove bay leaf and discard. Stir in parsley before serving.

Makes 4 servings.

ORANGE CHICKEN WITH ALMONDS

Fans of sweet-and-sour dishes will enjoy this orange-flavoured chicken. The almonds add calcium. Serve over basmati rice.

2	oranges
1 tbsp	canola oil
2	boneless skinless chicken breasts (4 oz each), diced
2 tsp	minced ginger root
1/4 tsp	each salt and freshly ground pepper
2	green onions, chopped
1	each red and green pepper, chopped
Pinch	red pepper flakes
1/4 cup	chicken stock (low-fat, low-sodium)
3 tbsp	soy sauce
2 tsp	cornstarch
1/2 cup	sliced almonds, toasted

1. Using rasp or grater, remove 1 tsp of the orange zest and set aside. Cut away orange zest and pith from 1 of the oranges and discard. Chop orange flesh coarsely. Cut other orange in half and squeeze out juice; set aside, discarding rind.
2. In large non-stick frying pan or wok, heat 1 1/2 tsp of the oil over medium-high heat. Cook chicken, ginger and a pinch each of the salt and pepper for about 6 minutes per side or until chicken is no longer pink inside. Transfer to plate. Add remaining oil to frying pan and cook green onions, red and green pepper, and red pepper flakes, stirring constantly, for about 6 minutes or until tender-crisp.
3. In small bowl, whisk together chicken stock, soy sauce, reserved orange zest and juice, cornstarch and remaining salt and pepper. Add chicken, chopped orange and vegetable mixture to frying pan and cook, stirring, for about 5 minutes or until sauce is thickened and chicken and vegetables are coated. Sprinkle with almonds and serve with rice.

Makes 2 servings.

CHICKEN TARRAGON WITH MUSHROOMS

Tarragon adds a light French flavour. The variation below is great for entertaining.

2 tsp	canola oil
2	boneless skinless chicken breasts (4 oz each)
	Freshly ground pepper
1 tsp	non-hydrogenated soft margarine
1	small onion, chopped
8 oz	mushrooms, sliced
3 tbsp	vermouth or white wine
1 tbsp	chopped fresh tarragon
½ cup	chicken stock (low-fat, low-sodium) or water

1. In non-stick frying pan, heat oil over medium-high heat. Sprinkle chicken with pepper and cook for about 6 minutes per side or until no longer pink inside. Transfer to plate and cover to keep warm.

2. Add margarine to frying pan and cook onion and mushrooms, stirring constantly, until soft, about 5 minutes. Add vermouth and tarragon, and simmer for 1 minute. Add stock and simmer for 2 minutes or until reduced by half. Season with pepper.

3. Serve sauce over chicken.

Makes 2 servings.

SPICY ROASTED CHICKEN WITH TOMATOES AND TARRAGON

This recipe is from our friend Meryle. Serve it with basmati rice or quinoa to soak up the sauce.

4 cups	cherry or grape tomatoes, halved
5	cloves garlic, crushed
¼ cup	extra-virgin olive oil
2 tbsp	chopped fresh tarragon
2 tsp	red pepper flakes
4	boneless skinless chicken breasts (4 oz each)
1 tsp	each salt and freshly ground pepper

1. Preheat oven to 450°F.

2. In large bowl, toss tomatoes with garlic, oil, 1 tbsp of the tarragon, and red pepper flakes.

3. Place chicken on rimmed baking sheet. Arrange tomato mixture in single layer around chicken. Sprinkle chicken and tomato mixture with salt and pepper. Roast for 30 to 35 minutes or until chicken is no longer pink inside. Transfer chicken to platter. Spoon tomatoes and juices over chicken and sprinkle with remaining tarragon.

Makes 4 servings.

ZESTY BARBECUED CHICKEN

The marinade in this recipe helps keep the breasts moist when they are cooked.

¼ cup	lemon juice
2 tsp	chopped fresh rosemary
2 tsp	canola oil
4	boneless skinless chicken breasts (4 oz each)
⅓ cup	Zesty Barbecue Sauce (see below)

1. In bowl, whisk together lemon juice, rosemary and oil. Add chicken breasts; toss to coat. Marinate at room temperature for 30 minutes.

2. Meanwhile, preheat oiled grill to medium-high.

3. Remove chicken from marinade and discard marinade. Brush chicken with Zesty Barbecue Sauce; grill for 6 minutes. Turn, brush with more sauce and grill for another 6 minutes or until chicken is no longer pink inside.

Makes 4 servings.

ZESTY BARBECUE SAUCE
This sauce will keep up to 2 weeks refrigerated in an airtight container.

1	can (398 mL) tomato sauce
2	cloves garlic, minced
¼ cup	frozen apple juice concentrate
¼ cup	tomato paste
2 tbsp	cider vinegar
1 tbsp	Splenda
1 tbsp	Dijon mustard
2 tsp	chili powder
½ tsp	Worcestershire sauce
¼ tsp	each salt and freshly ground pepper

1. In large saucepan, combine tomato sauce, garlic, apple juice concentrate, tomato paste, vinegar, Splenda, mustard, chili powder, Worcestershire sauce, salt and pepper; bring to boil. Reduce heat and simmer, uncovered, for about 20 minutes or until reduced and thickened.

Makes about 1 1/2 cups.

Meat

MEATLOAF

1 1/2 lbs	extra-lean ground beef
1 cup	tomato juice
1/2 cup	old-fashioned rolled oats (uncooked)
1	omega-3 egg, lightly beaten
1/2 cup	chopped onion
1 tbsp	Worcestershire sauce
1/2 tsp	salt (optional)
1/4 tsp	freshly ground pepper

1. Preheat oven to 350°F.

2. In large bowl, combine beef, tomato juice, oats, egg, onion, Worcestershire sauce, salt (if using) and pepper. Mix lightly but thoroughly.

3. Press meatloaf mixture into an 8- by 4-inch loaf pan. Bake for 1 hour, or until an instant-read meat thermometer inserted into the centre registers 160°F. Let meatloaf stand for 5 minutes before draining off any juices and slicing.

Makes 6 servings.

HORSERADISH BURGERS

The combination of beef and horseradish makes these burgers a hit with meat lovers.
For a spicier horseradish flavour, simply smother the top with some more horseradish.

1	small onion, grated
1	clove garlic, minced
2 tbsp	horseradish
2 tbsp	steak sauce
1 tbsp	Dijon mustard
1 tbsp	Worcestershire sauce
2 tbsp	chopped fresh oregano
1/4 tsp	salt
1/2 tsp	freshly ground pepper
2 tbsp	wheat bran
2 tbsp	wheat germ
1 lb	extra-lean ground beef
2	whole wheat buns, halved
4	leaves lettuce
1	tomato, sliced
1/4 cup	alfalfa sprouts (optional)

1. In large bowl, stir together onion, garlic, horseradish, steak sauce, mustard, Worcestershire sauce, oregano, salt and pepper. Add bran and wheat germ; stir to coat. Let stand for 5 minutes. Using hands, mix in beef until mixture is well combined.

2. Preheat oiled grill (optional). Form meat mixture into 4 patties about 1/2 inch thick. Place on grill or in non-stick frying pan and grill or cook, turning once, for about 12 minutes, or until no longer pink inside. Place patties on bun halves. Top with lettuce, tomato slices and sprouts (if using).

Makes 4 servings.

BEEF AND EGGPLANT CHILI

The addition of eggplant gives this chili a delicious twist. Sprinkle with low-fat Monterey Jack cheese for extra zip.

12 oz	extra-lean ground beef
1 tbsp	canola oil
2	onions, chopped
4	cloves garlic, minced
2 tbsp	chili powder
1 tbsp	dried oregano
1 tsp	ground cumin
2	green peppers, chopped
2 cups	diced eggplant
1	can (796 mL) diced tomatoes
½ cup	tomato paste
1	can (540 mL) red kidney beans, drained and rinsed

1. In large saucepan over medium-high heat, brown beef; remove to plate. In same saucepan, heat oil over medium heat. Cook onions, garlic, chili powder, oregano and cumin, stirring, for about 5 minutes or until softened. Add peppers and eggplant; cook for 10 minutes or until eggplant is lightly golden. Add tomatoes, tomato paste and browned beef; bring to boil. Reduce heat and add beans. Simmer for about 1 hour or until eggplant is very tender.

Makes 4 servings.

RIGATONI WITH MINI MEATBALLS

For busy families, a little meal preplanning always helps during the week. This hearty casserole can be made ahead of time and frozen for another day.

8 oz	lean ground chicken or turkey
2 tbsp	chopped fresh flat-leaf parsley
1	large clove garlic, minced
1 tsp	salt
Pinch	freshly ground pepper
1 tbsp	extra-virgin olive oil
1	onion, chopped
2 cups	chopped eggplant
1	zucchini, chopped
1	small carrot, finely chopped
1 tbsp	dried oregano
2	cans (796 mL each) plum tomatoes, puréed
1/2 cup	cooked red kidney beans
3 cups	rigatoni pasta
2 tbsp	grated Parmesan cheese

1. Preheat oven to 350°F.

2. In bowl, mix together chicken, parsley, garlic, and a pinch of the salt and pepper until well combined. Using wet hands, roll 1 heaping tsp of the mixture into a small meatball and place on parchment paper–lined baking sheet. Repeat with remaining mixture. Bake for about 8 minutes or until no longer pink inside.

3. Meanwhile, in large saucepan, heat oil over medium-high heat. Cook onion and eggplant, stirring, for about 8 minutes, or until golden and softened. Reduce heat to medium and add zucchini, carrot and oregano. Cook, stirring, for about 5 minutes or until softened. Add puréed tomatoes and remaining salt; bring to boil. Add cooked meatballs and beans; reduce heat and simmer for about 30 minutes or until sauce is slightly thickened.

4. Meanwhile, in large pot of boiling salted water, cook rigatoni for about 10 minutes or until al dente. Drain and add to meatballs and sauce; stir to combine. Sprinkle with Parmesan cheese.

Makes 4 to 6 servings.

PORK MEDALLIONS DIJON

Eating the green-light way doesn't mean you have to sacrifice flavour. This pork is fork-tender, and the tasty sauce is rich and creamy.

2	pork tenderloins (about 12 oz each)
5 tbsp	whole wheat flour
3/4 tsp	each salt and freshly ground pepper
2 tbsp	extra-virgin olive oil
2	onions, thinly sliced
1	clove garlic, minced
1/4 cup	Dijon mustard
1 1/4 cups	skim milk
1/2 cup	dry white wine
1 tbsp	chopped fresh tarragon

1. Slice pork into 3/4-inch medallions. Place between 2 pieces of waxed paper; using meat mallet or rolling pin, pound to about 1/4-inch thickness.

2. On dinner plate, combine 3 tbsp of the flour and 1/2 tsp each of the salt and pepper; dredge pork. In large non-stick frying pan, heat 1 tbsp of the oil over medium-high heat. Cook pork until golden brown on both sides, 5 to 7 minutes; transfer to the plate and cover to keep warm.

3. In same frying pan, heat remaining oil over medium heat. Cook onions and garlic, stirring often, for 5 minutes or until softened. Reduce heat to medium-low; cook, stirring occasionally, for 10 minutes or until golden. Add remaining flour and stir to coat onion. Add mustard; cook for 2 minutes. Stir in milk, wine and remaining salt and pepper. Cook, stirring constantly, until thickened. (If mixture is too thick, stir in 1 tbsp warm water.) Stir in tarragon. Return pork to pan and cook until heated through, about 1 minute.

Makes 6 servings.

MUSHROOM AND GRAVY PORK CHOPS

Nothing turns food into comfort food better than gravy. For a change, substitute chicken for pork chops.

1 tsp	dried Italian seasoning
½ tsp	dried basil
½ tsp	each salt and freshly ground pepper
4	boneless pork loin chops
2 tsp	extra-virgin olive oil
1	large onion, thinly sliced
1 lb	mushrooms, sliced
1 tbsp	chopped fresh thyme
2 tbsp	whole wheat flour
1 cup	chicken stock (low-fat, low-sodium)

1. In small bowl, combine Italian seasoning, basil, and ¼ tsp each of the salt and pepper. Sprinkle evenly on both sides of pork chops.

2. In large non-stick frying pan, heat oil over medium-high heat. Brown chops on both sides; transfer to plate and cover to keep warm. Add onion, mushrooms, thyme and remaining salt and pepper to the pan. Cook, stirring, for 10 minutes. Sprinkle with flour and cook, stirring, for 1 minute. Pour in stock, stirring to combine, and bring to boil. Reduce heat and simmer for about 3 minutes or until slightly thickened. Return pork chops to frying pan and cook, turning occasionally, for about 5 minutes or until just a hint of pink remains inside pork.

Makes 4 servings.

PORK TENDERLOIN WITH APPLE COMPOTE

Serve this comforting dish with Brussels sprouts, sliced carrots and some boiled new potatoes tossed in lemon juice and parsley.

1 tbsp	Dijon mustard
1/2 tsp	dried sage
1/4 tsp	dried thyme
Pinch	each salt and freshly ground pepper
1	pork tenderloin (about 12 oz)
1 tbsp	canola oil

Apple Compote:

1 tsp	canola oil
2	small apples, cored and diced
1	onion, finely chopped
1/4 tsp	dried thyme
Pinch	each salt and freshly ground pepper
1/4 cup	currants
2 tbsp	apple juice

1. Preheat oven to 400°F.

2. In small bowl, stir together mustard, sage, thyme, salt and pepper. Rub mixture all over tenderloin.

3. In ovenproof non-stick frying pan, heat the 1 tbsp oil over medium-high heat. Brown tenderloin on one side, turn over and place frying pan in oven for about 20 minutes or until pork has only a hint of pink inside. Let stand for 5 minutes before slicing.

4. **Apple Compote:** Meanwhile, in another non-stick frying pan, heat the 1 tsp oil over medium-high heat. Cook apples, onion, thyme, salt and pepper for 5 minutes or until light golden. Add currants and apple juice; cook for 1 minute or until apples are tender-crisp. Slice tenderloin and serve with Apple Compote.

Makes 3 servings.

Snacks

CRUNCHY CHICKPEAS

This is an addictive snack with all the crunch and saltiness of chips and pretzels but without the fat!

2	cans (540 mL each) chickpeas, drained and rinsed
2 tbsp	extra-virgin olive oil or canola oil
½ tsp	salt
Pinch	cayenne pepper

1. Preheat oven to 400°F.
2. In large bowl, toss chickpeas with oil, salt and cayenne. Spread on large baking sheet in a single layer.
3. Bake for about 45 minutes or until golden, shaking pan a couple of times during cooking. Let cool completely.

Makes 6 servings.

Helpful Hint: Add more salt or other spices to change the flavour of the chickpeas.

CRANBERRY CINNAMON BRAN MUFFINS

These muffins are very nutritious with a high fibre content and have a great cinnamon flavour.

1 cup	wheat bran
½ cup	All-Bran or 100% Bran cereal
¼ tsp	salt
½ cup	boiling water
1 cup	skim milk
1 cup	dried cranberries
⅓ cup	Splenda
1	omega-3 egg
¼ cup	canola oil
1 ¼ cups	whole wheat flour
1 ¼ tsp	baking soda
1 tsp	ground cinnamon

1. Preheat oven to 375°F. Line a 12-cup muffin tin with paper or foil liners.
2. In bowl, combine bran, cereal and salt. Pour boiling water over and stir to combine. Stir in milk and cranberries and set aside.
3. In another bowl, whisk together Splenda, egg and oil. Stir into bran mixture.
4. In large bowl, stir together flour, baking soda and cinnamon. Pour bran mixture over flour mixture and stir until just combined.
5. Divide batter among muffin cups. Bake for about 20 minutes or until tester inserted in centre of muffin comes out clean.

Makes 12 muffins.

Make Ahead: These muffins can be kept at room temperature for about 2 days or frozen for up to 1 month. (Wrap each muffin individually before freezing to help prevent freezer burn. Then place them in a resealable plastic bag or airtight container.)

CARROT MUFFINS

These healthful muffins are a delightful source of fibre.

1 cup	whole wheat flour
½ cup	wheat bran
½ cup	ground flaxseed
¼ cup	Splenda
2 tsp	baking powder
½ tsp	baking soda
2 tsp	ground cinnamon
1 tsp	ground ginger
¼ tsp	salt
1 cup	buttermilk
½ cup	liquid egg
¼ cup	canola oil
1 tsp	vanilla
1 ½ cups	finely grated carrot
½ cup	raisins, softened in hot water for 10 minutes and drained
⅓ cup	chopped pecans

1. Preheat oven to 375°F. Line a 12-cup muffin tin with paper or foil liners.
2. In large bowl, combine flour, bran, flaxseed, Splenda, baking powder, baking soda, cinnamon, ginger and salt.
3. In small bowl, whisk together buttermilk, liquid egg, oil and vanilla. Stir in carrot, raisins and pecans. Add flour mixture and stir just until combined.
4. Divide batter among muffin cups. Bake for 20 to 25 minutes or until tester inserted in centre of muffin comes out clean.

Makes 12 muffins.

Make Ahead: See page 279.

APPLE BRAN MUFFINS

Ruth created this recipe several years ago when I was trying to lose weight. We would make large batches and freeze them. Then, whenever I needed a snack, I'd warm one in the microwave. They were so convenient and delicious.

3/4 cup	All-Bran or Bran Buds cereal
1 cup	skim milk
2/3 cup	whole wheat flour
1/3 cup	Splenda
2 tsp	baking powder
1/2 tsp	baking soda
1/4 tsp	salt
1 tsp	ground allspice
1/2 tsp	ground cloves
1 1/4 cups	oat bran
2/3 cup	raisins
1	large apple, peeled and cut into 1/4-inch cubes
1	omega-3 egg, lightly beaten
2 tsp	canola oil
1/2 cup	unsweetened applesauce

1. Preheat oven to 350°F. Line a 12-cup muffin tin with paper or foil liners.

2. In a bowl, combine cereal and milk; let stand for a few minutes.

3. In large bowl, stir together flour, Splenda, baking powder, baking soda, salt, allspice and cloves. Stir in oat bran, raisins and apple.

4. In small bowl, combine egg, oil and applesauce. Stir, along with cereal mixture, into dry ingredients.

5. Divide batter among muffin cups. Bake until lightly browned, about 20 minutes.

Makes 12 muffins.

Make Ahead: See page 279.

WHOLE WHEAT FRUIT SCONES

Enjoy these scones with a hot cup of tea. They are even better with a little sugar-free fruit spread.

1 1/2 cups	whole wheat flour
1/2 cup	oat bran
1/2 cup	chopped dried apricots or dried cranberries
2 tbsp	Splenda
2 tsp	baking powder
1/2 tsp	salt
1/4 tsp	ground nutmeg
1/4 cup	non-hydrogenated soft margarine
2/3 cup	skim milk
2 tbsp	liquid egg

1. Preheat oven to 425°F.
2. In large bowl, combine flour, oat bran, dried apricots, Splenda, baking powder, salt and nutmeg. Using your fingers, rub margarine into flour mixture to combine. Add milk and toss with fork to form soft dough.
3. Place dough on floured surface and knead gently about 5 times. Pat dough out to 1/2-inch thickness. Cut dough into 8 squares, or use cookie or biscuit cutter to cut scones.
4. Place on baking sheet and brush tops with liquid egg. Bake for about 12 minutes or until golden on bottom.

Makes 8 scones.

STRAWBERRY TEA BREAD

This recipe makes two loaves, one for now and one for the freezer. A slice makes a perfect snack or a delicious dessert paired with sliced berries.

1 ½ cups	whole wheat flour
1 ½ cups	rolled oats
½ cup	wheat bran
1 tsp	cinnamon
1 tsp	baking soda
½ tsp	baking powder
½ tsp	salt
¾ cup	liquid egg
¾ cup	Splenda
½ cup	canola oil
½ cup	skim milk
1 tsp	vanilla
4 cups	strawberries, fresh or frozen and thawed, mashed

1. Preheat oven to 375°F. Oil two 9- by 5-inch loaf pans.

2. In large bowl, stir together flour, oats, bran, cinnamon, baking soda, baking powder and salt; set aside.

3. In separate bowl, whisk together liquid egg, Splenda, oil, milk and vanilla. Pour over dry ingredients and stir just until moistened. Stir in strawberries.

4. Divide mixture evenly between pans. Bake for 45 to 50 minutes or until cake tester inserted in centre comes out clean. Let cool in pan on rack for 15 minutes. Turn out onto rack and let cool completely.

Makes 2 loaves, 14 to 16 slices each. One serving is 1 slice.

Make Ahead: Wrap in plastic wrap or foil and store at room temperature up to 3 days, or wrap in plastic wrap and heavy-duty foil and freeze up to 1 month.

Desserts

BERRY CRUMBLE

This is one of Ruth's favourite green-light desserts. Though it's best made with fresh berries during the summer, it's also lovely with frozen fruit.

5 cups	fresh or frozen berries, such as raspberries, blackberries, blueberries and sliced strawberries
1	large apple, cored and chopped
2 tbsp	whole wheat flour
2 tbsp	Splenda
1/2 tsp	ground cinnamon

Topping:

1 cup	large-flake oats
1/2 cup	chopped pecans or walnuts
1/4 cup	brown Splenda
1/4 cup	non-hydrogenated soft margarine, melted
1 tsp	ground cinnamon

1. Preheat oven to 350°F.

2. In 8-inch square baking dish, combine berries and apple.

3. In bowl, combine flour, Splenda and cinnamon. Sprinkle over fruit and toss gently.

4. **Topping:** In medium bowl, combine oats, pecans, brown Splenda, margarine and cinnamon. Sprinkle over fruit mixture. Bake for about 30 minutes or until fruit is tender and top is golden.

Makes 6 servings.

Variation: Prepare as above and microwave on High for about 6 minutes or until fruit is tender. The top won't get golden or crisp in the microwave.

PLUM CRUMBLE

Crumbles are an ideal green-light dessert and can be made with a wide array of fruit.
Try using pears instead of the plums, cutting back slightly on the amount of Splenda.

1 ½ lbs	prune plums (such as damson or Italian), halved and pitted
1 tbsp	Splenda
1 tbsp	cornstarch
½ tsp	ground ginger
½ tsp	ground cinnamon

Topping:

3/4 cup	large-flake oats
½ cup	whole wheat flour
½ cup	Splenda
¼ cup	chopped almonds or pecans
¼ cup	non-hydrogenated soft margarine
1 tsp	grated orange zest
½ tsp	ground cinnamon
¼ tsp	ground cardamom

1. Preheat oven to 350°F.

2. In bowl, toss plums with Splenda, cornstarch, ginger and cinnamon. Arrange evenly in deep 9-inch pie plate.

3. **Topping:** In bowl, combine oats, flour, Splenda, almonds, margarine, orange zest, cinnamon and cardamom. Using your fingers, rub ingredients together until crumbly dough forms. Sprinkle evenly over fruit mixture. Bake for 35 to 40 minutes or until topping is golden and fruit mixture is bubbling.

Makes 6 servings.

Make Ahead: Refrigerate up to 2 days.

APPLE RASPBERRY COFFEE CAKE

A piece of this fruit-laden cake makes a delectable light dessert. It can be refrigerated for up to 3 days.

1 cup	whole wheat flour
1/2 cup	wheat bran
1/2 cup	brown Splenda
1 1/2 tsp	baking powder
1/2 tsp	baking soda
1/4 tsp	ground cinnamon
1/4 tsp	ground nutmeg
Pinch	salt
1/2 cup	buttermilk
1/4 cup	non-hydrogenated soft margarine, melted and cooled
1/4 cup	liquid egg
2 tsp	vanilla
1 cup	fresh raspberries
1	apple, cored and diced

Topping:

1/3 cup	large-flake oats
1/4 cup	brown Splenda
2 tbsp	chopped pecans
1 tbsp	non-hydrogenated soft margarine

1. Preheat oven to 350°F. Line an 8-inch square baking pan with parchment paper.

2. In large bowl, stir together flour, bran, brown Splenda, baking powder, baking soda, cinnamon, nutmeg and salt; set aside.

3. In another bowl, whisk together buttermilk, margarine, liquid egg and vanilla. Pour over flour mixture and stir until moistened. Spread two-thirds of the batter in prepared baking pan.

4. Toss raspberries and apple together and sprinkle over batter. Dollop with remaining batter, smoothly gently with wet spatula.

5. **Topping:** In bowl, combine oats, brown Splenda, pecans and margarine. Sprinkle over top of cake; press gently into batter. Bake for about 30 minutes or until tester inserted in centre comes out clean.

Makes 9 servings.

ONE-BOWL CHOCOLATE CAKE

This delicious cake is green-light when served with fresh berries. You can make a yellow-light version with chocolate ganache icing for a special occasion (see Variation below).

1 ¹/₃ cups	whole wheat flour
³/₄ cup	Splenda
¹/₂ cup	unsweetened cocoa powder
1 ¹/₂ tsp	baking soda
1 ¹/₂ tsp	baking powder
¹/₂ tsp	salt
1	omega-3 egg
1	omega-3 egg white
²/₃ cup	buttermilk
¹/₂ cup	unsweetened applesauce
2 tbsp	canola oil
1 tsp	vanilla
	Grated zest of 1 orange

1. Preheat oven to 350°F. Oil an 8-inch round cake pan or springform pan. Cut a round of parchment paper and line bottom of pan.

2. In mixer, food processor or blender, mix flour, Spenda, cocoa, baking powder, salt, egg, egg white, buttermilk, applesauce, oil, vanilla and orange zest just until smooth.

3. Pour batter into prepared pan, smoothing top. Bake for 20 to 25 minutes or until top springs back when lightly touched and tester inserted in centre comes out clean.

4. Let cool in pan on rack for 30 minutes. Remove from pan and remove parchment paper; let cool completely on rack.

Makes 8 servings.

Ganache variation: Melt 8 ounces of 70 percent chocolate in a bowl set over barely simmering water. Remove from heat and whisk in 1 ¹/₄ cups low-fat soy milk until smooth. Spread ganache over top and sides of cake.

APPLE PIE COOKIES

These cookies combine all the flavours of traditional apple pie and have a texture like a soft granola bar. A great snack.

1 cup	large-flake oats
3/4 cup	whole wheat flour
1 tsp	ground cinnamon
1/2 tsp	baking powder
Pinch	each ground nutmeg and salt
3/4 cup	unsweetened applesauce
1/3 cup	Splenda
1/3 cup	liquid egg
2 tsp	vanilla
1	apple, cored and finely diced

1. Preheat oven to 275°F. Line baking sheet with parchment paper.
2. In large bowl, combine oats, flour, cinnamon, baking powder, nutmeg and salt.
3. In separate bowl, whisk together applesauce, Splenda, liquid egg and vanilla. Pour over oats mixture and stir to combine. Add apple and stir to distribute evenly.
4. Drop by heaping tablespoonfuls onto prepared baking sheet. Bake for about 25 minutes or until firm and lightly golden. Let cool completely.

Makes about 18 cookies. One serving is 1 cookie.

Make Ahead: Store in airtight container up to 3 days or freeze up to 2 weeks.

PECAN BROWNIES

Brownies, you ask? That's right. These are packed with fibre and are absolutely scrumptious, so get baking!

1	can (540 mL) white or red kidney or black beans, drained and rinsed
½ cup	skim milk
⅓ cup	liquid egg
¼ cup	non-hydrogenated soft margarine, melted
1 tbsp	vanilla
¾ cup	Splenda
½ cup	whole wheat flour
½ cup	unsweetened cocoa powder
1 tsp	baking powder
Pinch	salt
½ cup	chopped toasted pecans

1. Preheat oven to 350°F. Line an 8-inch square baking pan with parchment paper.
2. In food processor, purée beans until coarse. Add milk, liquid egg, margarine and vanilla, and purée until smooth, scraping down sides a few times. Set aside.
3. In large bowl, combine Splenda, flour, cocoa, baking powder and salt. Pour bean mixture over flour mixture and stir to combine. Scrape batter into prepared pan, smoothing top. Sprinkle with pecans.
4. Bake for about 18 minutes or until tester inserted in centre comes out clean. Let cool on rack, then cut into 16 squares.

Makes 16 brownies. One serving is one brownie.

Make Ahead: Wrap brownies in plastic wrap or store in an airtight container for up to 4 days. They can also be frozen for up to 2 weeks.

CREAMY LEMON SQUARES

These tiny treats make an ideal mid-afternoon pick-me-up.

½ cup	whole wheat flour
½ cup	wheat bran
¼ cup	ground almonds
¼ cup	Splenda
¼ cup	non-hydrogenated soft margarine

Filling:

1 cup	Splenda
3/4 cup	liquid egg
2 tsp	grated lemon zest
½ cup	fresh lemon juice
¼ cup	buttermilk
2 tsp	cornstarch
1 tsp	baking powder

1. Preheat oven to 350°F. Oil an 8-inch square baking pan.
2. In mixer or food processor, combine flour, bran, almonds and Splenda. Cut in margarine until mixture is crumbly.
3. Press mixture evenly into bottom of prepared pan. Bake for 20 to 25 minutes or until lightly browned. Set aside to cool, leaving oven on.
4. **Filling:** In bowl, whisk together Splenda and liquid egg. Stir in lemon zest and juice, buttermilk, cornstarch and baking powder. Pour over base. Bake for 15 to 20 minutes or until filling is set. Let cool to room temperature, then refrigerate for at least 2 hours before cutting into squares.

Makes 36 squares. One serving is 2 squares.

Make Ahead: Store in airtight container up to 3 days or freeze up to 1 month.

Appendix

Complete G.I. Diet Food Guide

BEANS

Baked beans with pork	Baked beans* (low fat)
Broad	Black beans
Refried	Black-eyed peas
	Butter beans
	Chickpeas
	Italian
	Kidney
	Lentils
	Lima
	Mung
	Navy
	Pigeon
	Refried (low fat)
	Romano
	Soybeans
	Split peas

* Limit serving size to ¹/₂ cup.

BEVERAGES

Alcoholic drinks*	Diet soft drinks (caffeinated)	Bottled water
Cocout milk	Milk (1%)	Club soda
Fruit drinks	Most unsweetened juice	Decaffeinated coffee (with skim milk, no sugar)
Milk (whole or 2%)	Red wine*	Diet soft drinks (no caffeine)
Regular coffee	Vegetable juices	Herbal tea
Regular soft drinks		Light instant chocolate
Rice milk		Milk (skim)
Sweetened juice		Soy milk (plain, low fat)
Watermelon juice		Tea (with skim milk, no sugar)

BREADS

Bagels	Crispbreads (with fibre)*	100% stone-ground whole wheat*
Baguette/Croissants	Pita (whole wheat)	Crispbreads (with high fibre, e.g., Wasa Fibre)*
Cake/Cookies	Tortillas (whole wheat)	
Cornbread	Whole-grain breads	Whole-grain, high-fibre breads (2½ to 3 g fibre per slice)*
Crispbreads (regular)		
Croutons		
English muffins		
Hamburger buns		
Hot dog buns		
Kaiser rolls		
Melba toast		
Muffins/Doughnuts		
Pancakes/Waffles		
Pizza		
Stuffing		

* Limit serving size (see page 21).

Tortillas

White bread

CEREALS

All cold cereals except those listed as yellow- or green-light	Kashi Go Lean Crunch	100% Bran
Cereal/Granola bars	Kashi Good Friends	All-Bran
Granola	Shredded Wheat Bran	Bran Buds
Grits		Cold cereals with minimum 10 g fibre per serving
Muesli (commercial)		Fibre 1
		Fibre First
		Kashi Go Lean
		Oat Bran
		Porridge (large flake oats)
		Red River

CEREAL/GRAINS

Amaranth	Cornstarch	Arrowroot flour
Almond flour	Spelt	Barley
Couscous	Whole wheat couscous	Buckwheat
Millet		Bulgur
Polenta		Gram flour
Rice (short-grain, white, instant)		Kamut (not puffed)
Rice cakes		Quinoa
Rice noodles		Rice (basmati, wild, brown, long-grain)
		Wheat berries

CONDIMENTS/SEASONINGS

Croutons	Mayonnaise (light)	Capers
Ketchup		Chili powder
Mayonnaise		Extracts (vanilla, etc.)
Tartar sauce		Garlic

		Gravy mix (maximum 20 calories per ¼ cup serving)
		Herbs
		Horseradish
		Hummus
		Mayonnaise (fat-free)
		Mustard
		Salsa (no added sugar)
		Sauerkraut
		Soy sauce (low sodium)
		Spices
		Teriyaki sauce
		Vinegar
		Worcestershire sauce

DAIRY

Almond milk	Cheese (low fat)	Buttermilk
Cheese	Cream cheese (light)	Cheese (fat-free)
Chocolate milk	Frozen yogurt (low fat, low sugar)	Cottage cheese (1% or fat-free)
Coconut milk	Ice cream (low fat)	Cream cheese (fat-free)
Cottage cheese (whole or 2%)	Milk (1%)	Extra low-fat cheese (e.g., Laughing Cow Light, Boursin Light)
Cream	Sour cream (light)	
Cream cheese	Yogurt (low fat, with sugar)	Fruit yogurt (non-fat with sweetener)
Evaporated milk		
Goat milk		Ice cream (½ cup, low-fat and no added sugar, e.g., Breyers Premium Fat Free, Nestlé Legend)
Ice cream		
Milk (whole or 2%)		
Rice milk		
Sour cream		

Yogurt (whole or 2%)		Milk (skim)
		Sour cream (fat-free)
		Soy milk (plain, low fat)
		Soy cheese (low fat)

FATS AND OILS

Butter	Corn oil	Almonds*
Coconut oil	Mayonnaise (light)	Canola oil*/seed
Hard margarine	Most nuts	Cashews*
Lard	Natural nut butters	Flax seed
Mayonnaise	Natural peanut butter	Hazelnuts*
Palm oil	Peanuts	Macadamia nuts*
Peanut butter (regular and light)	Pecans	Mayonnaise (fat-free)
Salad dressings (regular)	Salad dressings (light)	Olive oil*
	Sesame oil	Pistachios*
Tropical oils	Soft margarine (non-hydrogenated)	Salad dressings (low fat, low sugar)
Vegetable shortening	Soy oil	Soft margarine (non-hydrogenated, light)*
	Sunflower oil	Vegetable oil sprays
	Vegetable oils	
	Walnuts	

FRUITS

FRESH

Cantaloupe	Apricots	Apples
Honeydew melon	Bananas	Avocado* (¼)
Kumquats	Custard apples	Blackberries
Watermelon	Figs	Blueberries
	Kiwi	Cherries
	Mango	Cranberries
	Papaya	Grapefruit
	Persimmon	Grapes
	Pineapple	Guavas

* Limit serving size (see page 13).

Cantaloupe	Pomegranates	Apples
Honeydew melon		Nectarines
Kumquats		Lemons
Watermelon		Nectarines
		Oranges (all varieties)
		Peaches
		Plums
		Pears
		Raspberries
		Rhubarb
		Strawberries

BOTTLED, CANNED, DRIED, FROZEN

All canned fruit in syrup	Canned apricots in juice or water	Applesauce (without sugar)
Applesauce containing sugar	Dried apples	Frozen berries
Most dried fruit** (including dates and raisins)	Dried apricots**	Fruit spreads with fruit, not sugar as the main ingredient
	Dried cranberries**	Mandarin oranges
	Fruit cocktail in juice	Peaches/Pears in juice or water
	Peaches/Pears in syrup	

JUICES*

Fruit drinks	Apple (unsweetened)	
Prune	Cranberry (unsweetened)	
Sweetened juice	Grapefruit (unsweetened)	
Watermelon	Orange (unsweetened)	
	Pear (unsweetened)	
	Pineapple (unsweetened)	
	Vegetable	

* Whenever possible, eat the fruit rather than drink its juice.
** For baking, it is OK to use a modest amount of driedapricots or cranberries.

Beef (brisket, short ribs)	Beef (sirloin steak, sirloin tip)	All fish and seafood, fresh, frozen or canned (in water)
Bologna	Chicken/Turkey leg (skinless)	Back bacon
Breaded fish and seafood	Corn beef	Beef (top/eye round steak)
Duck	Dried beef	Chicken breast (skinless)
Fish canned in oil	Flank steak	Egg whites
Goose	Ground beef (lean)	Ground beef (extra lean)
Ground beef (more than 10% fat)	Lamb (fore/leg shank, centre cut loin chop)	Lean deli ham
Hamburgers	Pork (centre loin, fresh ham, shank, sirloin, top loin)	Liquid eggs (e.g., Break Free)
Hot dogs	Turkey bacon	Moose
Lamb (rack)	Whole omega-3 eggs	Pastrami (turkey)
Organ meats	Tofu	Pork tenderloin
Pastrami (beef)		Sashimi
Pâté		Soy/Whey protein powder
Pork (back ribs, blade, spare ribs)		Soy cheese (low fat)
Regular bacon		Tofu (low fat)
Salami		Turkey breast (skinless)
Sausages		Turkey roll
Sushi		TVP (Textured Vegetable Protein)
Whole regular eggs		Veal
		Veggie burger
		Venison

PASTA

All canned pastas		Capellini
Gnocchi		Fettuccine
Macaroni and cheese		Macaroni
Noodles (canned or instant)		Mung bean noodles
		Penne
Pasta filled with cheese or meat		Rigatoni
Rice noodles		Spaghetti/Linguine
		Vermicelli

PASTA SAUCES

Alfredo	Sauces with vegetables (no added sugar)	Light sauces with vegetables (no added sugar, e.g., Healthy Choice)
Sauces with added meat or cheese		
Sauces with added sugar or sucrose		

SNACKS

Bagels	Bananas	Almonds*
Candy	Dark chocolate* (70% cocoa)	Applesauce (unsweetened)
Cookies	Ice cream (low fat)	Canned peaches/pears in juice or water
Crackers	Most nuts*	
Doughnuts	Popcorn (air-popped microwaveable)	Cottage cheese (1% or fat-free)
Flavoured gelatin (all varieties)		Extra low-fat cheese (e.g., Laughing Cow Light, Boursin Light)
French fries		
Ice cream		Fruit yogurt (non-fat with sweetener)
Muffins (commercial)		Food bars*
Popcorn (regular)		Hazelnuts**
Potato chips		Ice cream (1/2 cup, low fat and no added sugar, e.g., Breyers Premium Fat Free)
Pretzels		
Pudding		
Raisins		

* 180–225 calorie bars, e.g., Zone or Balance Bars; 1/2 bar per serving
* * Limit serving size (see page 13).

Rice cakes		Most fresh fruit
Sorbet		Most fresh vegetables
Tortilla chips		Most seeds
Trail mix		Pickles
White bread		Sugar-free hard candies

SOUPS

All cream-based soups	Canned chicken noodle	Chunky bean and vegetable soups (e.g., Campbell's Healthy Request, Healthy Choice)
Canned black bean	Canned lentil	
Canned green pea	Canned tomato	
Canned puréed vegetable		Homemade soups with green-light ingredients
Canned split pea		

SPREADS & PRESERVES

All products that have sugar as the first ingredient listed	Fructose	Fruit spreads (with fruit, not sugar, as the first ingredient)
	Sugar alcohols	Marmite

SUGAR & SWEETENERS

Corn syrup	Fructose	Aspartame
Glucose	Sugar alcohols	Equal
Honey		Splenda
Molasses		Stevia (note: not FDA approved)
Sugar (all types)		Sugar Twin
		Sweet'N Low

Broad beans	Artichokes	Alfalfa sprouts	Cauliflower
French fries	Beets	Asparagus	Celery
Hash browns	Corn	Beans (green/wax)	Collard greens
Parsnips	Potatoes (boiled)	Bell peppers	Cucumbers
Potatoes (instant)	Pumpkin	Bok choy	Eggplant
Potatoes (mashed or baked)	Squash	Broccoli	Fennel
Rutabaga	Sweet potatoes	Brussels sprouts	Hearts of palm
Turnip	Yams	Cabbage (all varieties)	Kale
		Carrots	Kohlrabi
		Mustard greens	Leeks
		Okra	Lettuce
		Olives*	Mushrooms
		Onions	Radicchio
		Peas	Radishes
		Peppers (hot)	Rapini
		Pickles	Snow peas
		Potatoes (boiled, new small)*	Spinach
			Swiss chard
			Tomatoes
			Zucchini

* Limit serving size (see page 13).

Acknowledgements

I owe a special debt to Stacey Cameron at Random House, who has edited all six of my books to date. Her help and guidance in bringing order to the mountain of feedback from Clinic participants was invaluable. She truly brought the book to life.

My wife, Ruth, Professor Emeritus at the University of Toronto and an authority on changing behaviours, provided penetrating insights into the emotional and behavioral challenges faced by Clinic members. She was also responsible for the recipe selection, as she has been for the entire G.I. Diet series. I could not ask for a better partner both professionally and personally.

Index

goose, 291
grains
    charts, 26, 31, 35, 287
    overconsumption, 9
gram flour, 287
granola, 26, 287
granola bars, 287
grapefruit, 26, 31, 35, 289
grapefruit juice, 27, 290
grapes, 26, 31, 35, 289
gravy mix, 288
grazing, 78, 122
green-light foods
    adjusting recipes, 68–69
    Phase I, 21
    Phase II, 198–99
    Preliminary Phase, 21
    preparing your kitchen, 46
    role, 17
    shopping for, 46–47
grits, 287
guavas, 289

H
habits
    cleaning the plate, 80
    eating high-sugar, high-fat treats, 81
    eating too quickly, 78–79
    grazing, 78
    not drinking enough, 79
    not taking time to eat properly, 77–78
    recognizing, 78–79
    rewarding exercise, 79–80
    shopping on empty stomach, 80–81
    skipping breakfast, 76–77
    unconscious eating, 78
ham, lean deli, 25, 30, 34, 291
hamburger buns, 31, 286
hamburgers
    charts, 30, 34, 99, 291
    from fast food restaurants, 99–101
    homemade, 37
Harvey's, 101
hash browns, 27, 294
hazelnuts, 27, 36, 40, 289, 292
health

disease risks of excess weight, 14, 45, 56,
    151–52, 153–54
    and weight loss, 56–57
heart disease
    and carbohydrates, 8
    and fats, 10–11
    and weight, 45, 56, 150–51, 154
hearts of palm, 294
herbs, 288
hiking, 172
holidays, 81, 143, 160–63
honey, 293
honeydew melons, 289
horseradish, 288
hot dog buns, 31
hot dogs, 30, 34, 291
hummus, 288
hypertension, 151, 153

I
ice cream, 40, 288, 292
indoor activities, 173–75
insulin, 15–16

J
jams, 29, 290, 293
Jenkins, David, 14
jogging, 172
joint degeneration, 154
juices
    complete G.I. diet chart, 290
    sweetened, 27, 286, 290
    unsweetened, 27, 286
    vegetable, 286

K
Kaiser rolls, 286
kale, 294
kamut, 287
Kashi
    Go Lean cereal, 26, 287
    Go Lean Crunch cereal, 26, 287
    Good Friends cereal, 26, 287
ketchup, 287
kiwis, 26, 31, 35, 289
kohlrabi, 294

kumquats, 289

L

labels, 47
lamb
    lean cuts, 30, 34, 291
    rack, 291
lard, 289
leeks, 31, 35, 294
lemons, 31, 35, 290
lentils, 285
lettuce, 31, 35, 294
lunch
    carbohydrates, 31–32
    fats, 32
    in Phase II, 199
    proteins, 30
    salads, 33
    sandwiches, 33
    soups, 32

M

macadamia nuts, 289
macaroni and cheese, 31, 35, 292
mangoes, 26, 31, 35, 289
margarine
    hard, 11, 27, 32, 36, 289
    soft
        non-hydrogenated, 27, 32, 36, 289
        non-hydrogenated, light, 27, 29, 32,
            36, 289
marmite, 293
mayonnaise
    fat-free, 32, 36, 288, 289
    light, 32, 36, 287, 289
    regular, 32, 36, 287, 289
McDonald's, 99
meal basics
    about, 24–25
    breakfast, 25–30
    dinner, 33–39
    lunch, 30–33
    snacks, 39–40
meal planning
    week 2, 66–67
    while travelling, 103

meats
    at restaurants, 97–98
    complete G.I. diet chart, 291
    fat content, 11
    for breakfast, 25
    for dinner, 34, 36, 37
    for lunch, 30
    processed, 30, 34
    protein content, 12
melba toast, 286
melons, 26, 31, 35, 289
men
    appropriate BMI, 44
    waist measurement, 45, 153–54
menopause, 132
milk
    1%, 25, 34, 286, 288
    almond, 288
    buttermilk, 25, 288
    chocolate, 288
    coconut, 288
    evaporated, 288
    goat, 288
    rice, 286, 288
    skim, 25, 29, 34, 41, 289
    soy, 25, 34, 286, 289
    whole or 2%, 25, 29, 34, 286, 288
millet, 287
minerals, 8
molasses, 293
moose meat, 291
motivation, 139–44
muesli, commercial, 26, 287
muffins
    commercial, 35, 40, 292
    complete G.I. chart, 286
    green-light, 26
    red-light, 26, 31
mushrooms, 32, 35, 294
mustard, 288
mustard greens, 294

N

nectarines, 290
noodles
    canned or instant, 31, 35, 292

air-popped, 40, 292
regular, 40, 292
pork
back ribs, blade or spare ribs, 291
lean cuts, 30, 34, 291
porridge see oats
potato chips, 40, 292
potatoes
at restaurants, 97
boiled, 31, 32, 35, 36, 294
French fries, 27, 31, 35, 40, 292, 294
glycemic index, 17
hash browns, 27, 294
holiday dinners, 161
instant, 294
mashed or baked, 31, 35, 294
serving size, 38
sweet, 32, 35, 161, 294
poultry
at restaurants, 97–98
complete G.I. diet chart, 291
for dinner, 34, 36, 37
for lunch, 30
protein content, 12
Preliminary Phase
green-light foods, 21
serving sizes, 20–21, 24
what to eat, 20
when to eat, 24
prepared foods, 9
preserves, 293
President's Choice Blue Menu jams, 29
pretzels, 40, 292
processed foods, 9
processed meats, 30, 34
proteins
for breakfast, 25
for dinner, 34
for lunch, 30
and green-light recipes, 69
role, 12
sources, 12
prune juice, 27, 290
pudding, 40, 292
pumpkin, 294

pumpkin seeds, 40

Q
quinoa, 31, 35, 287

R
radicchio, 294
radishes, 32, 36, 294
raisins, 40, 290, 292
rapini, 294
raspberries, 32, 36, 290
recipes see also separate recipe index
adjusting to green-light, 68–69
maximizing cooking time, 69
Red River Cereal, 26, 287
red-light foods, avoiding, 17
restaurants, 96–106
rhubarb, 290
rice
basmati, wild, brown or long-grain, 31, 35, 287
glycemic index, 17
serving size, 38
short-grain, white or instant, 31, 35, 287
rice cakes, 40, 287, 293
rice milk, 286, 288
rice noodles, 287, 292
rutabagas, 31, 294

S
salad dressings
from fast food restaurants, 99–102
light, 32, 36, 289
low fat, low sugar, 32, 36, 289
regular, 32, 36, 289
salads
at restaurants, 97, 99
for lunch, 33
from fast food restaurants, 99–102
holiday dinners, 161
salami, 291
salsa, 288
sandwiches
from fast food restaurants, 99–102
green-light, 33
sashimi, 291

appropriate BMI, 44
emotional eating, 120
menopause, 132
plateaus, 132
waist measurement, 45, 153–54
worcestershire sauce, 288

Y
yams, 32, 35, 294
yellow-light foods, role, 17
yoga, 175
yogurt

frozen, low fat, low sugar, 288
fruit, non-fat with sugar substitute, 25,
    29, 34, 40, 288, 292
low fat, with sugar, 25, 34, 288
whole or 2%, 25, 34, 289

Z
zucchini, 32, 36, 294

Recipe Index

Italian Omelette, 210
Mini Breakfast Puffs, 208
Vegetarian Omelette, 211
Western Omelette, 212

F
Fettucine Primavera, 231
Fish see also specific fish
    G.I. Fillet, 244
    Pan-Seared, with Mandarin Salsa, 248
French Toast, Cinnamon, 206

G
Ganache, 281
G.I. Fish Fillet, 244
G.I. Pasta Salad, 225
G.I. Salad, Basic, 221
G.I. Vinaigrette, Basic, 221
Ginger-Wasabi Halibut, 246
Greek Salad, 223
Grilled Tuna with Chimichurri Sauce, 247

H
Haddock, Citrus-Poached, 245
Halibut, Ginger-Wasabi, 246
Ham
    Ham and Lentil Soup, 217
    Western Omelette, 212
Homey Oatmeal, 204
Horseradish Burgers, 262

K
Kale, Tuscan White Bean Soup, 215

L
Lasagna, Easy-Bake, 237
Leeks
    Barley Risotto with Leeks, Lemon and
        Peas, 232
    Vegetable Crumble, 233
Lemons
    Barley Risotto with Leeks, Lemon and
        Peas, 232
    Creamy Lemon Squares, 284
Lentils, Ham and Lentil Soup, 217
Lettuce

Basic G.I. Salad, 221
iceberg, Greek Salad, 223
romaine, Caesar Salad, 222

M
Mandarin Salsa, 248
Meatloaf, 261
Minestrone Soup, 214
Mixed Bean Salad, 227
Moussaka, Vegetarian, 239
Muesli, Homemade, 205
Muffins see Breads and Muffins
Mushrooms
    Chicken Tarragon with Mushrooms, 256
    Italian Omelette, 210
    Mushroom and Gravy Pork Chops, 267
    Vegetable Crumble, 233
    Vegetarian Omelette, 211

N
Nuts
    almonds, Orange Chicken with Almonds, 255
    mixed, Vegetable Crumble, 233
    pecans
        Apple Raspberry Coffee Cake, 279
        Berry Crumble, 277
        Carrot Muffins, 272
        Pecan Brownies, 283
        Plum Crumble, 278
    walnuts
        Berry Crumble, 277
        Waldorf Chicken and Rice Salad, 228

O
Oats
    Apple Pie Cookies, 282
    Apple Raspberry Coffee Cake, 279
    Berry Crumble, 277
    Homemade Muesli, 205
    Homey Oatmeal, 204
    Meatloaf, 261
    Oatmeal Buttermilk Pancakes, 207
    Plum Crumble, 278
    Strawberry Tea Bread, 275
Olives, Greek Salad, 223
Omelettes